The
Brain Food
Diet

About the author

A consultant physician with more than thirty years' experience in medicine, Dr Frank Ryan is a Fellow of the Royal
College of Physicians, the Royal Society of Medicine and
the Linnean Society of London. He is also a distinguished
author, whose books have been acclaimed worldwide and
translated into many languages. *Tuberculosis: The Greatest
Story Never Told* was 'Book of the Year' for the *New York
Times* and *Darwin's Blind Spot* was the 'Chosen Book' for
the celebrated financial expert Charlie Munger.

The Eskimo Diet, which Frank co-authored with Dr Reg
Saynor, began the omega-3 revolution and was a bestseller
in the UK.

Other books by Frank Ryan
Non-fiction

The Eskimo Diet (co-author Reg Saynor)
Virus X
Darwin's Blind Spot
Tuberculosis: The Greatest Story Never Told (in the US, *The
Forgotten Plague*)

Fiction

Between Clouds and the Sea

The
Brain Food
Diet

How to stay young in mind with
the omega-3s

DR FRANK RYAN

P

PROFILE BOOKS

First published in Great Britain in 2007 by
Profile Books Ltd
3a Exmouth House
Pine Street
Exmouth Market
London EC1R 0JH
www.profilebooks.com

10 9 8 7 6 5 4 3 2 1

A CIP catalogue record fo
British Library.

ISBN 978 1 84668 098 4

Text design by Sue Lamble
Typeset in Stone Serif by MacGuru Ltd
info@macguru.org.uk

Printed and bound in the UK by
CPI Bookmarque, Croydon, CR0 4TD

Disclaimer
This publication is intended to provide helpful and informative
material on the subjects addressed. It is sold with the understanding
that the authors and publisher are not engaged in rendering medical,
health or any other kind of personal professional services in the book.
The authors and publisher specifically disclaim all responsibility for
any liability, loss, or risk, personal or otherwise, which is incurred as a
consequence, directly or indirectly, of the use and application of any of
the contents of this book

Contents

Acknowledgements

I would like to thank Ginny Rose for her prompting, which led me to write this book. I would further like to thank her for her helpful reading and suggestions for clarification. I am also indebted to my editor, Daniel Crewe, for his advice and encouragement, to my agent, Jonathan Pegg, for his indefatigable support and dedication, and to my wife, Barbara, for reading the script and correcting my cookery transgressions.

Declare the past, diagnose the present, foretell the future.
Hippocrates of Cos, *Epidemics*, Book 1, section 11

*I wish this book, as the child of my brain, to be the most
beautiful, the liveliest and cleverest possible.
But I have been unable to transgress the order of nature by
which like gives birth to like.*
Cervantes, *Don Quixote*

For Pat

Author's note

This book does not promise miracle cures or a replacement for any treatment that you may already be taking. All I ask is that you consider the facts, which I will present in plain, simple English, and then decide for yourself if your diet is deficient in the marine omega-3 fatty acids. If, like most people in the UK, your diet does lack these essential ingredients, I shall show you how, in the simplest possible way, you can rebalance your diet and reduce the risk of the mental decline that is mistakenly assumed to be a part of normal ageing.

I shall also show you how to plan your daily diet so that you get the right balance between the omega-3s and omega-6s – a balance that is now known to be highly important. This is the first time, to my knowledge, that this balance has been explained to the public. But if you have any special concerns about eating fish, or taking cod liver oil or fish oil, you should take the advice of your doctor.

Those looking for more detailed medical advice or scientific information will find a guide to further reading at the end of this book, together with a free, comprehensive source of advice, information and references at www.swiftpublishers.com.

Introduction

Gimme that zing

Do you have days when you wake up feeling good about yourself, days when that inner sun is shining? When there is a ready smile on your face when you greet people, a youthful zing about you – so much so that everybody wants to know what's making you feel so good? Well, today I want to help you recapture a little of that zing. And the reason I can say this with some confidence is because I have a scientifically proven message to give you, an important message that will enable you to help yourself.

'What will it cost me?' I hear you ask.

I can assure you that the financial cost is very little. And if you anticipate that the cost will be paid in terms of punishment, frugality, starvation or a fad diet, or doing without the things you love – those little things that make your life worthwhile – then the answer is nothing at all. You see my message really is a happy one. It will not interfere with your quality of life, except perhaps to make it better.

Remember that one universal truth we all grasped a long time ago? The one thing we can count on is the fact that we are getting older every day. That worries some of us, I know. There are aspects of it that worry me too. Some people get themselves into a tizzy and go to extreme lengths to try to ward off the effects of ageing. Nobody wants to slow down, get wrinkly and frayed around the edges, creak in the joints and, worst of all, become forgetful and slow mentally. In fact, when it comes down to it, that's what we fear more than anything – that we'll lose that zing. There's a medical term for it, 'age-related cognitive decline', or ARCD, which in essence means the progressive loss of the ability to think, with its implicit erosion of memory and all of the important social graces and dignities that go with it.

Well, here's the good news: thanks to some very recent advances in medical knowledge, there really is something we can do to help ourselves.

Some of you might remember how this story began in 1990, when Reg Saynor and I co-authored *The Eskimo Diet*. This brought about a nutritional and medical revolution in the UK and Ireland. But at the time it was highly controversial. I was working as a consultant physician in a major teaching hospital, which was also the regional cardiac referral centre. I had twenty years' experience treating heart attacks, and indeed all of the common and serious medical conditions I shall be talking about in this book. Up to that point patients who had suffered heart attacks, or who were thought to be at high risk of a heart attack because they had angina or high cholesterol levels in their blood, were told to *avoid* oily fish. Reg had been running a blood fat clinic at the hospital for years and had pioneered the study of fish oil in treating abnormal blood fat levels. He believed he had more than enough evidence to prove the very opposite – that fish oil has properties that *reduce* blood fats and the risk of heart attacks. We combined our experience to write *The Eskimo Diet*, which caught the attention of the media and helped to change dietary habits for the better.

This was the beginning of the omega-3 story. Little did we realise that what we knew then, revolutionary as it seemed, was merely the tip of the iceberg in a remarkable chapter of discovery with major biological and medical implications, including human evolution, and diseases as varied as rheumatoid arthritis, lupus, schizophrenia and depression. We shall examine this story while focusing on one area in particular: how fish oil, and the omega-3s it contains, helps to slow down, and in some ways even prevent, memory loss and the other mental afflictions that we regard as the consequence of ageing. Indeed, fish oil and those remarkable omega-3s may also considerably reduce the risk of getting Alzheimer's disease. It may even help treat some people who have already developed a mild form of the disease. Moreover, there is growing evidence that it may help to lighten your mood.

So you see, it really is a zing thing.

These are major claims. How could a natural dietary ingredient do all of these things? This is such an important question it needs to be looked at closely, without hype or the rose-tinted spectacles of wishful thinking. Yet the exciting thing is that over the last few years this message has become increasingly credible through good quality scientific and medical research.

But I don't expect you to just take my word for it. In this book I invite you to join me on a wonderful voyage of discovery in which I shall set out the evidence in plain and simple language so you can make up your own mind. Then, assuming you are convinced, I shall show you how to modify your diet and lifestyle to put the zing back into your life.

The health-giving properties of the omega-3s

Old wives' tales, of course, had it that fish was good for the brain long before medical science took it seriously. But when *The Eskimo Diet* was first published, some of my colleagues were inclined to joke about codfathers and briny old tales of the sea. In fact, belief in the health-giving properties of fish oil is very ancient indeed. The Romans knew about it, as, very likely, did earlier folk. They noticed that fish oil was good for their health. And then, a couple of thousand years later, doctors became interested in rickets.

Rickets is a serious disease that stunts the growth and development of children. In the late nineteenth and early twentieth centuries it reached epidemic proportions in Northern Europe and America and as a consequence proved bad for army recruitment because 20–30 per cent of young men failed their medical due to the effects of childhood rickets. Something had to be done.

Rickets is caused by a lack of vitamin D. We manufacture vitamin D in our skin, under the beneficial action of direct sunlight. But in the cloudy and polluted atmosphere of the northern hemisphere, there isn't enough direct sunlight to make it happen. Knowing that cod liver oil is rich in vitamin D, the enlightened government health advisers set up health promotion programmes aimed at mums, with the message: Get your kids to take a spoonful of cod liver oil a day!

Mums got the message. Whole generations of children grew up with the taste of cod liver oil, often downed under threat or with the taste masked by malt or lemon. Moreover, it worked. The plague of childhood rickets was eradicated in a single generation. Cod liver oil and orange juice (for vitamin C) were also made available to children and pregnant women during the Second World War and the years of rationing that followed. And that was thought to be that. Nobody imagined there was more to the story until an Oxford don, Hugh Sinclair, took it into his head to prove otherwise.

Sinclair was in the best tradition of the dons of his day in combining intellectual brilliance with eccentricity. Fascinated by nutrition, in 1944 he travelled to Canada, where he took advantage of the opportunity to visit the Eskimos. These people, now known as Inuit, ate a diet so high in saturated fat it would give a cardiologist nightmares, yet they didn't appear to suffer from heart attacks. For Sinclair it was an enigma too provocative to be ignored. When he visited the Eskimos, he confirmed that they didn't appear to suffer from heart attacks and they lacked the tell-tale white ring on the outer margin of the iris, known as a premature *arcus senilis*, that can signal the presence of high blood fats.

In 1976, together with two Danish scientists, Dyerberg and Bang, Sinclair made a second trip to meet the Eskimos in Greenland. They found that the Eskimos' blood cholesterol levels were no different from our own. Furthermore, other blood fats called triglycerides, which are also linked to heart attacks, were much lower than they would have expected, given the Eskimos' high blubber diet. This really was perplexing. Sinclair could think of only two possible explanations: either the Eskimos had evolved to be resistant to the bad effects of a very high fat diet, or there was something in their diet that was protecting them.

Three years later he had the brainwave of putting himself on the Eskimo diet. He imported a whole seal, whose blubber would supply him with a high fat diet, and he otherwise ate nothing but fish and shellfish. I should point out that this is a good deal less balanced than the real diet of the Eskimos. Over three months or so, his weight fell by a couple of stones, though it's hardly a diet I would recommend for weight reduction. His blood fats also changed to mirror the pattern he had seen in the Eskimos, confirming that their perplexing blood fats were caused by their diet. But there was another, and wholly unpredicted, effect of this extreme marine diet. The clotting ability of his blood became seriously impaired, so much so he developed extensive bruising and blood appeared in his urine. This suggested that not only did a fishy diet improve blood fats it also reduced the risk of forming a blood clot – a major factor in heart attacks.

Sinclair's pioneering experiment would have monumental medical implications.

That same year, my colleague Reg Saynor saw Sinclair being interviewed on television. Reg, who ran the cardiothoracic laboratory at our hospital, was worried about his own abnormal blood fats. But instead of putting himself on Sinclair's extreme diet, Reg bought a bottle of cod liver oil. He soon discovered that a spoonful had much the same effects on his blood fats as Sinclair's diet, without being so extreme as to threaten his health. He then began a series of experiments, testing various types and doses of fish oil for their beneficial effects on cholesterol and triglycerides – and further in preventing heart attacks. All his experiments pointed to protection against heart attacks, even in patients with bad blood fats who had severe angina or who had already suffered a heart attack.

When Reg and I got together to write *The Eskimo Diet,* I added my experience in dealing with heart attacks and my knowledge of nutrition. In a later chapter, this story will be brought up to date and extended to the rainbow of benefits the omega-3s offer sufferers from many different illnesses. But it is time we returned to the all-important question of preventing unwanted memory loss and other indignities of ageing.

2

What the omega-3s really are

In *Gulliver's Travels* the Immortals of Luggnagg never bothered to read because their memories were so poor they had forgotten the beginning of a sentence before they got to the end. The author, Jonathan Swift, might have been describing Alzheimer's disease, that tragic affliction that affects increasing numbers of people living in the UK. Anything that reduces the risk of getting Alzheimer's disease, or that might help mitigate its effects, is worth knowing about. However, lesser Luggnaggian problems afflict most of us sooner or later – and long before what we would consider old age. We all have occasional embarrassing memory lapses, when we forget what we are shopping for or meet an acquaintance and can't recall his or her name.

The sad fact is that, sooner or later, many of us are destined to suffer the effects of age-related cognitive decline.

'Hey,' I hear you exclaim, 'I'm already halfway there!'

'Me too,' I have to admit, 'at times!'

But isn't there an important clue in that everyday observation?

On some days we feel less than sharp, while on other days we could shave the head off a pencil. The same is true with Alzheimer's disease, particularly in the early stages when the unfortunate sufferers have moments, or even days, when they appear to recover their faculties. The fluctuating nature of the illness suggests that whatever is blunting the clarity of memory and thinking may be treatable, particularly in the earlier stages.

Thank goodness memory lapses aren't permanent in our more mundane day-to-day fluctuations! How much more so does this fluctuating tendency apply to our moods, whether happy or sad. If a chemical change in our brain can influence memory, wit and even that elusive inner peace and happiness, it suggests that there may be ways in which we can influence our brain chemistry to improve and protect those blessings.

Even when *The Eskimo Diet* was first published we knew that the omega-3 fatty acids in fish oil play a role in the development and health of the brain. In the intervening years, and particularly in the last decade or so, the supportive evidence has become overwhelming. What, then, are the omega-3s, and why are they so important?

You can compare fatty acids to a string of beads made of carbon, with chemical links between each one. If all the links are single strands (a single bond), the fatty acid is called a saturated fat. If one of the links is a double strand (a double bond), it is called a monounsaturated fat, a good example of which is oleic acid. Olive oil, with its large amounts of oleic acid, is an integral part of the so-called Mediterranean diet, which reduces blood cholesterol and lessens the risk of suffering a heart attack. If two or more of the links in a fatty acid are double-stranded, it is called a polyunsaturated fat, or polyunsaturated fatty acid (PUFA). The fatty acids that are essential to human health – the so-called essential fatty acids (EFAs) – are PUFAs.

DHA is one of these, with no fewer than six double strands. Because the first of the double strands is on the third bead or carbon from the distant (omega) end of the string, it's called an omega-3 polyunsaturated fatty acid. Fat accounts for roughly 55 per cent of the substance of our brains, but this is a very special type of fat – not the kind we pile on our waists, hips and thighs. This so-called structural fat is an integral part of the membranes of the nerve cells. DHA is the main fatty acid found in these structures and it is especially concentrated in the vast proliferation of nerve-to-nerve junctions, known as synapses, that ramify throughout the cortex – the 'thinking part' of the brain. We know that deficiency of the omega-3s causes a reduction in the chemicals that transmit signals in these synapses, creating a demonstrable malfunction in some of the key brain pathways.

DHA is also a major component of the myelin sheath, which is wrapped like insulation around the long processes of nerves. Integrity of the myelin is of the utmost importance for normal brain function. Deficiency of omega-3s in the postnatal period leads to major delay in forming this insulation, leading to impaired learning, and motor, visual and auditory abnormalities. Inflammation and damage to myelin also plays an important part in multiple sclerosis.

The highest concentration of DHA is found in the retina – the light-sensitive lining at the back of the eyes – where it plays an important role in vision. In men it also plays a role in the tail-wagging movement, or motility, of the sperm.

Eicosapentaenoic acid (EPA) is another omega-3

polyunsaturated fatty acid, with five double strands in a slightly shorter string than DHA. EPA also plays an important part in the health of our heart and circulation, and is important in reducing inflammation.

It is important to grasp that DHA and EPA are only found in any significant quantity in marine foods, especially the edible flesh of oily fish, such as herrings, salmon and mackerel, and the livers of white fish, such as cod and haddock. Another important source of DHA, and the only significant vegetarian one, is certain marine algae, which provide the DHA that is now used to fortify bottled milk formulas.

There are two families of essential fatty acids: omega-6 and omega-3. Omega-6 linoleic acid (LA) is plentiful in plants, particularly their seeds. LA is readily converted to arachidonic acid (ARA) in the body. Arachidonic acid itself is also readily available from a normal diet, in meat, eggs and dairy produce. It's a moot point whether you regard linoleic acid as the essential fatty acid, or both linoleic acid and arachidonic acid. As you may have figured out, in ARA and LA the first double strand is on the sixth carbon from the distant, or omega, end of the string. Arachidonic acid also plays an important role in brain development and normal day-to-day functioning. But given the many sources of both these omega-6s in the diet, deficiency of ARA is unlikely in normal circumstances.

Alpha-linolenic acid (ALA) is an omega-3 fatty acid of plant origin, and it is found in flaxseeds, walnuts, soy nuts and soybean oil. It acts as a source of energy for the body and can be used as a building block for DHA and EPA. But this conversion process is slow and inefficient, with only 5–10 per cent of ALA being converted to EPA, and even less converted to DHA. This means that the only reliable way to get enough of these essential ingredients is to consume DHA and EPA. We face a simple choice – either we eat a meal of oily fish at least twice a week or we supplement our diet with a high quality omega-3 source, such as fish oil or a cod liver oil.

General symptoms of essential fatty acid deficiency include fatigue, skin and hair problems, and weakening of the immune system. The key question as far as this book is concerned is this: just how important are these omega-3 nutrients to our mental health?

In Bristol a far-sighted medical and nutritional team, based at the university, has been conducting a long-term study aimed at improving the health and development of children. Known as the 'Children of the 90s', they have examined the effects of diet on development.

Most of the baby's brain maturation takes place during the last three months of pregnancy and in the first two years of life. But, as you might imagine, it's difficult to measure brain development in such young infants. But one thing we can measure is their ability to recognise depth in three-dimensional images, an ability known as stereopsis. Using stereopsis as a test of general brain development, ophthalmic experts compared brain development in breast-fed and bottle-fed infants. They arrived at two separate and equally startling conclusions:

- **Children who were breast-fed for four months or more were more likely to have high-grade brain function.**

● **Children born to mums who ate oily fish were likely to have higher-grade brain function.**

These were far-reaching observations. Human breast milk contains omega-3 DHA but, until recently, milk formulas for bottle-feeding did not. So it was inevitable that breast-fed babies had higher levels of DHA in their brains than those who were bottle-fed. The Bristol results were confirmed by studies in other countries. Indeed, when the experts compared reading, visual interpretation, sentence completion and even mathematical ability, the breast-fed children performed better.

Some sceptics still argued that better performance didn't necessarily mean that omega-3s were the key ingredients. There were alternative explanations, like the fact breast-feeding is more often associated with higher socioeconomic class, and thus perhaps the breast-fed infants might have enjoyed a better general level of nutrition, and perhaps also better healthcare and welfare.

In Norway Helland and her colleagues put this possibility to the test. They studied the effects of two different food supplements in 590 pregnant and lactating mothers, giving half of them corn oil (vegetable-type omega-6) and the other half cod liver oil (omega-3 EPA and DHA). When they tested their babies, those with mothers given cod liver oil were larger and had better brain maturation at birth. Of course, babies' brains continue to develop after birth. However, when the same researchers conducted an IQ test on the same children at the age of four, they still found higher scores in those whose mothers had taken cod liver oil in pregnancy or during lactation. They now added a third important conclusion to the evolving story – in their words:

● **Maternal intake of [fish oil] during pregnancy and**
   lactation may be favourable for later mental
   development of children.

Ricardo Uauy, Professor of Public Health Nutrition at
the London School of Hygiene and Tropical Medicine,
went a step further. Comparing brain and eye function in
breast-fed babies and bottle-fed babies, he found that when
the bottle-fed babies received supplements of fish oil they
had the same scores as the breast-fed infants. He then
arrived at a fourth important conclusion:

● **The advantages of breast-fed over bottle-fed infants**
   were due to a better intake of omega-3 DHA and
   EPA.

The next question was fairly predictable. Did this
advantage stop after the breast-feeding stage?

In the USA, Birch and her colleagues looked at infant
brain development after the breast-feeding period, taking
as their measure the eyesight of 65 healthy babies who had
been weaned from the mother's milk at six weeks. They
were interested in the fact that the visual cortex, the part of
the brain responsible for sight, matures after the six-week
period. The infants were then divided into two groups.
One group was weaned on a standard formula feed, which
contained the vegetable omega-6 and vegetable omega-3
but contained no DHA, and the other group was weaned
on the same formula fortified with DHA. In spite of the fact
that both groups enjoyed a good supply of omega-3s from
the mothers' milk for the first six weeks, the infants who
were subsequently weaned on bottle milk not fortified with
DHA had significantly poorer eyesight than those given

DHA when eyesight was measured at 17, 26 and 52 weeks. In the experts' words, 'Better acuity at 52 weeks was correlated with higher concentrations of docosahexaenoic acid [DHA] in plasma and red blood cells.' They added a fifth important conclusion:

● **The fish type of omega-3s plays an important role in brain development and maturation long after birth.**

The implications were so important that Japanese health authorities, concerned about a possible intellectual decline in the population as result of switching from the traditional Japanese diet which is rich in seafood and vegetables to Western-style junk food, launched a campaign to increase the intake of omega-3s in Japanese children.

At this stage I should let Professor James A. McGregor, in his advice to American obstetricians, speak:

> [First-class scientific studies] have shown us that polyunsaturated fatty acids have the potential to improve pregnancy performance and measures of neurocognition in babies and children. The results of [these studies] suggest that both reduced rates of prematurity and increased childhood neurocognition can be provided by improving omega-3 fatty acid nutrition in pregnancy, lactation and early childhood.

McGregor also suggested that the mothers' own health would benefit from taking the right amount of omega-3s in their diets. McGregor went on to emphasise to his colleagues what he was recommending:

All sources of omega-3 fatty acids are not equal. Fish is the only source of easily available eicosapentaenoic acid (EPA) and DHA.

Mums who rarely or never eat oily fish or other rich marine sources should be concerned about these conclusions. This also applies to mums who are vegetarians if they assume that their bodies can convert the omega-3s found in vegetable sources to sufficient quantity of those that come exclusively from marine sources. In my former medical practice I investigated a great many vegetarians suffering from anaemia or from peripheral nerve damage. Most were suffering from iron deficiency (iron is mainly derived from meat and liver) or vitamin B12. This was long before I realised the importance of the omega-3s. Today, vegetarians tend to be better informed. If they haven't already done so, vegetarian readers should join the Vegetarian Society of the United Kingdom, which will give them advice on how to avoid all deficiency states, and in particular how to get hold of the essential omega-3s.

By now there is a large and growing library of information, derived from trials in many different countries, that confirms the importance of polyunsaturated fats – and omega-3 in particular – in the development of the infant's brain. Could it be that these same omega-3 fats also play a vital role in the health and function of our brains no matter what our age?

3

Omega-3s in our day-to-day mental function

In Shakespeare's *A Midsummer Night's Dream* Snug declares, 'Give it to me, for I am slow of study.' Well, who isn't, you might say! We associate memory decline with the passing of years, but while some slowing down is probably inevitable, memory loss that undermines our quality of life and health is not. I encountered much the same assumption after the *Eskimo Diet* was published, when some of my medical colleagues thought that heart attacks were a natural process in ageing. Nobody these days would regard heart attacks as part of normal ageing. We now know they are the result of disease. And this is exactly how we should regard age-related cognitive decline.

Indeed, the world of medicine might have been accused of being Snug's bedfellow when it came to appreciating the importance of the omega-3 fatty acids such as DHA and EPA. When you consider that the long chain fatty acids were found to be 'essential' to growth and health by the husband and wife team Burr and Burr as long ago as 1929, it has taken us rather a long time to wake up to their full nutritional role in our health and well-being. As a result of this, some colleagues still miss the central message of this book and assume that fish oil and the omega-3s should be treated as if they were drugs.

In fact, they're a normal and essential part of our diet. From an evolutionary point of view, it seems likely that our distant ancestors consumed fish and shellfish regularly, so that they became central to physical development and health. Indeed, in the opinion of Professor Crawford of the Institute of Brain Chemistry and Human Nutrition at the University of North London, the omega-3s may have played a central role in the evolution of the human brain. Whether we take them as fish, a cod liver oil supplement or an omega-3 supplement, we are not doing anything unnatural. Instead, we are restoring nutritional balance to our diet and helping to prevent developmental stagnation in infants as well as preventing illnesses in older children and adults which, in varying degree, result from a deficiency or lack of these essential nutrients.

In 1982 an American doctor, named Holman, reported the case of a six-year-old girl who had been shot in the stomach. Let's call her Jenny. Jenny's injury resulted in severe bowel damage and she had to be fed intravenously. By 1982 doctors knew that we need a regular intake of essential fats, but they were unaware that DHA and EPA were 'essential' in this strict medical sense. So Jenny's drip fluid was fortified with safflower oil, which is high in the omega-6 linoleic acid but almost devoid of omega-3s. After five months of drip-feeding Jenny developed numbness and tingling in her hands and feet, weakness in her legs and ultimately the inability to walk, blurred vision and psychological disturbance. These symptoms suggested brain and peripheral nerve damage. By now experts were beginning to realise the importance of omega-3 fatty acids so they checked Jenny's blood, and the results revealed gross omega-3 deficiency. When they swapped safflower oil for soybean oil, which provides omega-3 alpha-linolenic acid (ALA), the little girl's condition slowly returned to normal.

Today we would assume that the key deficiency was of EPA or DHA. As we saw earlier, the body can convert alpha-linolenic acid to EPA and DHA, albeit slowly and inefficiently. Had the doctors known this and given Jenny a fish oil supplement, her response might have been quicker. But this is not to detract from their very precious achievement, which was to save Jenny's life.

Of course, the rapid brain growth and development that takes place in the womb and extends into the first two years of life is long over in a child of six. Yet it would appear that the lack of omega-3s was still critical to the health of Jenny's brain and peripheral nervous system. Her story became a milestone in our understanding of the role of omega-3 fatty acids in day-to-day brain function and it triggered a great deal of research.

Even at the time Dr Holman was treating Jenny, tests were being conducted in laboratory rats and mice. It may strike some people as odd to test cognition in animals, but all mammals use problem-solving and learning behaviour in their efforts to find food and survive. The brains of rats and mice are made up of the same types of nerve cells and nerve junctions as the brain of humans, and omega-3 fats are the single most important component of the structural fats in their brains and in the back of their eyes. One of the reasons why Dr Holman tried omega-3 supplementation in Jenny's case was due to a test conducted in rats by Lamptey and Walker five years earlier. They fed safflower oil (high in omega-6 but low in omega-3) to one group of rats and a diet containing a good supply of omega-3 in the form of alpha-linolenic acid to another group. When they compared the rats' performance in finding their way out of a maze, rats fed exclusively omega-6 found their way out of the maze 60 per cent of the time, whereas those fed omega-3s found the way out 90 per cent of the time.

Since then a range of tests have been conducted in rats, mice and baboons, confirming that omega-3s really do enhance problem-solving performance. When the diets of animals are deficient in omega-3s, problem-solving and learning ability fall dramatically. And yes, you might have guessed it, they have even looked at the effects of omega-3s in older rats.

Ageing in rats is, of course, relative. Two years in a rat's life equates to pensionable age in humans. In a study conducted by Gamoh and colleagues in Japan, the administration of DHA to 'older' rats significantly improved tests of memory, including working memory – or at least what passes for it in rats. The question, then, is this: Do these tests on brain function in animals really mean the same to you and me?

We've seen how important omega-3 fatty acids are to the developing foetus and the newborn when the brain is very actively growing and developing. And in Jenny's case, we saw how it remains important long after the brain had gone through its phase of rapid growth and development. In the mid-1990s, Stephens and colleagues at Purdue University, Indiana wondered if omega-3 fatty acid deficiency might play a part in attention deficit hyperactivity disorder (ADHD), a condition in which children are unusually inattentive, impulsive and hyperactive. When they measured blood concentrations of three essential fatty acids, the omega-6 arachidonic acid and the omega-3s DHA and EPA, they found a significant association between ADHD and low blood levels of all three.

Just because these levels are low in ADHD, it doesn't necessarily follow that this is the cause of the condition. Even today the cause of ADHD remains elusive, but it is likely that it is caused by several different factors, so a single line of therapy is unlikely to work for all affected children. Nevertheless, when the same group treated the children with omega-3 supplementation, their parents and teachers reported some improvement in their behaviour.

The same group also studied learning problems in 100 boys aged 6–12. They found that the children with the highest levels of omega-3 fatty acids in their blood had the fewest learning difficulties.

In the UK, Richardson and her colleagues found evidence that dietary fatty acid deficiency or imbalances may contribute to the severity of dyslexia, while also contributing to dyspraxia (which results in poor coordination and delayed speech), ADHD and autism. In the USA, Zhang and colleagues looked at whether polyunsaturated fat deficiency might be linked to abnormal behaviour and learning difficulties. When they analysed the diets of 3,666 children aged 6–16 and measured achievement and IQ, the total dietary fat intakes had no significance, but when they looked at polyunsaturated fats there appeared to be a dose-related link between poor intake of polyunsaturated fats and poor performance.

Dose-linked findings like this are very suggestive. However, the polyunsaturated fatty acids were not broken down into the various omega types, nor were blood levels of omega-3 taken, so their impact could not be measured.

So what about adults – and in particular adults over the age of 50? Do these remarkable findings in children hold true in maturity?

One way in which you can measure the efficiency of brain function is to look at the transmission of brainwave patterns during tests of learning and memory. The faster the brainwave is transmitted, the more efficiently the brain is working. The rate of transmission declines with age and it is significantly slower in people with dementia. After an initial set of tests, 26 healthy adults were given supplements of either DHA or EPA and retested. Just two hours after taking DHA, they showed a significant improvement of their brainwave patterns. This suggests that DHA has an almost immediate effect on brain chemistry, a role that would appear to be different from its effect on brain development in infants. This fits with the evidence from other animal studies in which DHA has been shown to help in signalling between nerve cells in the brain.

When I was a medical student, I was taught that our brain cells stop dividing in our youth, leading to a progressive fall in the number of cells in the brain. This, it was thought, explained mental decline as people aged. In fact, we now know that the picture is far more complex. Adult brain cells do have some capacity to divide. And of vital importance is the potential to set up new and better connections between different brain cells, and between different parts of the brain as a whole. This function remains highly active into old age.

In adults the effects of DHA are not just immediate or short term. One of the interesting results of the studies in animals was the fact that it took at least a month for mice fed DHA supplementation to make significantly fewer mistakes working their way through a maze – and by this time the supplemented older animals performed even better than younger ones whose diet did not contain DHA. This could not have resulted from rapid changes in nerve chemistry as seen in the human volunteers in the brainwave experiment. It suggests additional applications and nerve pathways where DHA may be important.

This leads us to the key question. Will supplementing our diet with omega-3s protect us from the mental decline that people assume is part of the process of ageing?

4

Preventing cognitive decline

In 2000, William E. Connor, working at the Health Sciences University in Portland, Oregon, wrote an important review paper titled 'Importance of n-3 fatty acids in health and disease'. He began with this statement:

> In the past 2 decades, views about dietary n-3 [omega-3] fatty acids have moved from speculation about their functions to solid evidence that they are not only essential nutrients but also may favourably modulate many diseases.

Connor's review introduced a supplement of the *American Journal of Clinical Nutrition*, which contained no fewer than 38 studies on the importance of omega-3 fatty acids in health and disease. Clearly, the subject was now of intense interest. Several of the articles suggested that not only was deficiency of particular omega-3s a key element in a number of common and serious diseases, such as heart attacks, lupus and rheumatoid arthritis, but also that *an increased ratio of omega-6s to omega-3s* in the diet could accentuate the risk. It is important to grasp this key concept, since omega-6s and omega-3s may exert very different effects

– for example, an imbalance towards omega-6s may promote chemical pathways that give rise to inflammation, whereas omega-3s tend to promote pathways that control inflammation.

Our bodies will usually obtain a plentiful supply of the vegetable omega-3 alpha-linolenic acid (ALA), from dietary sources. But the ALA in our body has to compete with the omega-6s for access to the chemical mechanisms necessary to convert this to the fish-type omega-3s, EPA and DHA. Thus the typical Western diet, which tends to be skewed towards omega-6s, impairs the already very inefficient natural conversion of ALA to EPA and DHA. This imbalance has become all the more relevant because in our world, with its hustle and bustle and over-reliance on processed oils and convenience foods, increased consumption of vegetable oils rich in omega-6, such as arachidonic and linoleic acids, has coincided with a reduced consumption of the omega-3s, DHA and EPA.

This is not to say that omega-6 fatty acids are harmful. Linoleic acid and arachidonic acid are also essential nutrients and play key roles in the healthy function of our brain. One of my patients took dietary fads to extremes, believing that all fats, even vegetable oils, were bad for him. He ended up eating no fat at all. By the time I saw him, which was only a few months into his idiosyncratic diet, his skin was dry and flaking, his hair was falling out and he was so weak he could hardly rise from a chair. Had he continued on this diet, the hazards would have been extreme. The advice, of course, is not to avoid any one type of fat, but to get the balance right. Later in this book I'll give some practical guidance on how to achieve this, but now I need to return to the more general discussion.

The bulk of Connor's review is devoted to a summary of the importance of omega-3s in heart disease and brain development in infancy, reflecting the fact that in 2000 this was the front line. As we have seen, breast milk always contains DHA. But only a year earlier, Artemis P. Simopoulos, nutritional adviser to the Office of Consumer Affairs at the White House, drew attention to the fact that US manufacturers of baby food were not required to add DHA to their products. So, even as recently as 2000, it wasn't unreasonable to give priority to the need for infant brain development. But studies of the potential benefit of marine-derived omega-3s in adults were already underway.

Before we look at some important studies of fish and omega-3 intake in relation to mental decline, there are a few general points we need to consider.

Population studies looking at dietary influence on health are notoriously difficult to conduct because there are a great many variables that have to be taken into account. Different researchers adopt various yardsticks – some look closely at diet and may go so far as to analyse local fish for omega-3 content. Others don't look at diet at all, but measure different types of blood fats, whether in the plasma or in the membranes of red cells. To add to this, intake of foods other than those under scrutiny may also influence the outcome, as may smoking and alcohol consumption. Other complicating factors include intelligence and education, which may influence food choices, and other aspects of lifestyle, such as obesity and exercise. More subtle still is the influence of culture. Lifestyles and diet vary enormously between cultures, for example between Japan and the USA, and between both Japan and the USA and the European states. And even within Europe we are familiar with huge differences in diet and lifestyle between, say, the UK and the Mediterranean countries. So it is with a certain degree of caution that we shall take a look at the findings of some important studies from around the world.

Some of these difficulties were addressed by Whalley and his colleagues at the University of Aberdeen, who reported in the *American Journal of Nutrition* in 2004. Taking as their starting point the assumption that mental performance in later life is affected by environmental factors during our lifetime, they set out to discover if food supplements affected the mental decline associated with ageing. They began by highlighting a common and important criticism of any such study: what if only a certain kind of person takes omega-3 supplements? To play devil's advocate, what if the kind of person who takes omega-3 supplements is smarter than average to begin with?

A nationwide questionnaire sent to women in Norway had suggested exactly this. Roughly 45 per cent of the women who responded took cod liver oil regularly and these women were more likely to have a higher education, be physically active and have less tendency to obesity. Critics could now suggest that when we compare supplement-takers with non-takers, what we're really comparing is a smarter and more health-conscious subset of the population and not the effects of taking omega-3s at all.

Whalley was able to answer this question because the Scottish Council for Research in Education had previously tested the IQs of children born in 1936 and tested in 1947. The same people could now be studied in old age.

They focused on children born in Aberdeen and randomly selected a group of 423 men and women, all of whom agreed to be examined. Of these about 350 completed the study, with roughly equal numbers of men and women. At the time of testing they were all aged 64. Questioning included occupational history, consumption of alcohol, smoking, a detailed medical history, height and weight, detailed dietary habit assessment, and assessments for dementia through verbal learning tests, IQ testing and various other tests of mental ability. A dietary assessment was complemented by blood tests, which allowed a detailed breakdown of different fat intakes, including saturated fat, polyunsaturated fat, and omega-9, omega-6 and omega-3 fatty acids.

Whalley and colleagues arrived at a number of interesting conclusions. As expected, women were more likely to take supplements than men. But there were no links between supplement-takers or non-takers when it came to occupation, obesity, smoking or alcohol consumption. While there was an association between fish oil supplement-takers and higher levels of childhood IQ, they were now able to correct for this by selecting equivalent IQ subsets and thus arrive at their findings.

Did taking fish oil do people any good? In the experts' own summary:

> Food supplement use and [red blood cell] omega-3 content are associated with better cognitive ageing. If associations with omega-3 content are causal, optimization of omega-3 and omega-6 fatty acid intakes could improve retention of cognitive function in old age.

A year later, Morris and her colleagues reported a large community study of residents of Chicago, aged 65 and over, in which they examined whether fish and omega-3 fatty acids affected age-related mental decline. Their conclusions were curiously contradictory in that they found that fish intake was indeed associated with less mental decline, but, although there was a suggestion that this was linked to omega-3s, they were unable to pin this down with estimations of the omega-3 intakes in the diet. This was puzzling – indeed, it contradicted their own earlier study in which they observed strong reductions in Alzheimer's disease among people who had high intakes of omega-3s. Although they speculated on why this might be, they could offer no definite explanation.

There were other contradictory studies. In 2003 Laurin and her colleagues reported negative findings from the Canadian Study in Health and Ageing, a trial based on 18 research centres throughout Canada. They looked at people aged 65 and over and compared those with cognitive impairment and dementia to people with normal mental ability, and measured the levels of various fats in the plasma part of the blood. Unlike most other studies, they found higher levels of EPA in the plasma of cognitively impaired people, and higher DHA levels and polyunsaturated fats in those with dementia. They concluded that omega-3s did *not* protect people from cognitive decline or dementia.

Some aspects of the Canadian study are open to criticism. Although the study grew as an offshoot of long-term observation of very large numbers of people, those participating were gradually whittled down to just 174, of whom 79 had normal function with 43 cognitively impaired and 52 having dementia. These numbers suggest very small samples from each participating centre, a factor that may have skewed their attempts at a random mix. Moreover, they made no attempt to assess whether the test population had Alzheimer's disease or any other cause of dementia.

Like some of the other studies, they made no attempt to collect dietary information, but relied on plasma levels of fatty acids from a single venous blood sample taken after a meal, with some of the samples being stored for lengthy periods. Unfortunately, many of their test population were also institutionalised, a situation likely to have profound effects on dietary and other factors.

A previous Canadian study by Conquer and her colleagues had examined the plasma levels of omega-3s in 84 elderly people, comparing normals with those suffering cognitive impairment, Alzheimer's disease and other dementias. This study also relied on blood levels of fatty acids rather than dietary histories and suffered from the fact there were relatively small numbers in the test population, but their findings contradicted those of Laurin and her colleagues. Conquer and colleagues found low levels of DHA in both the cognitively impaired and the Alzheimer group, while the total omega-6 levels were significantly higher in both groups. They concluded that low blood levels of omega-3 may be a risk factor for both cognitive impairment and Alzheimer's disease.

How are we to make sense of the fact that two studies from the same country have drawn entirely opposite conclusions?

There is a clear need to study larger numbers of people over as long a period as possible, the test subjects possessing normal cognition to start with, and living freely in the community so that they control their own diets and lifestyles.

A study of this nature was in fact conducted at the National Institute of Health and Medical Research, in Ville-juif, France, under the guidance of Heude and her colleagues. The same researchers had been examining a large group for arterial disease over many years – the so-called EVA Study. In 1995 they extended this to include mental decline, measuring both the initial cognitive ability as well as the fatty acid composition of the blood in 246 men and women aged between 63 and 74. This gave them both a normal cognitive starting point and an objective measure of the long-term dietary consumption of various types of fatty acids. Over four years of follow-up, they continued to assess the mental ability of these subjects to see if there was any relationship between the degree of cognitive decline and the levels of the different types of fatty acid in the blood. They also took into account age, gender, smoking habits, alcohol consumption, history of heart disease, objective measures of arterial disease, blood pressure, body mass index and education level.

Their technique of measuring fatty acids in the blood was different from earlier studies. Rather than take a one-off measure of the fatty acids in the liquid, or plasma, part of the blood, they measured the fatty acid levels in red cell membranes, which might give a better indication of long-term dietary intakes.

Their study revealed 'significant differences in fatty acid composition between the decline and no-decline groups'. Higher levels of saturated fat and omega-6 unsaturated fatty acids were associated with greater risk of mental decline. Higher levels of omega-3 fatty acids were associated with a lesser tendency to mental decline. In their conclusions, they suggested that, while these results required confirmation by other researchers, here was a new rationale for studying how these *modifiable* risk factors might be implicated in the cognitive ageing process. By 'modifiable' they implied that, if their results were confirmed, they offered a means of prevention or possible treatment.

In the April 2007 issue of *The American Journal of Clinical Nutrition,* two groups of researchers confirmed the French workers' conclusions in prospective trials. The first of these was a multi-centre study conducted by Beydoun and colleagues at the University of North Carolina, the School of Public Health, University of Minnesota, Minneapolis, and the Center for Human Nutrition, Johns Hopkins School of Public Health, Baltimore. This study also grew out of a previous population study of arterial disease, the Atherosclerosis Risk in Communities (ARIC) Study, which had been monitoring fatty acids in white residents of Minneapolis from 1987.

From 1990 to 1992, and again from 1996 to 1998, they conducted tests of mental function in 2,251 men and women residing in Minneapolis, in whom the fatty acid levels in the blood plasma were also recorded. Known as the Minneapolis Study, the test population differed from the French group in including much larger numbers of people. They also extended the age of their test population to include younger people, beginning at the baseline of 50–65 years. To my mind, this is sensible as I suspect that cognitive decline may begin long before pensionable age. If that's true, then prevention should also start earlier. They found an increased risk of overall cognitive decline in those with high levels of palmitic acid and omega-6 arachidonic acid (ARA), but the risk was reduced in those with higher concentrations of linoleic acid, another omega-6 fatty acid. They found no clear link between omega-3 levels and overall cognitive decline. But when they focused on verbal fluency, a key facet of mental capability, they found the higher the plasma levels of DHA and EPA the less cognitive decline. This protection was most obvious in people who also suffered from high blood pressure or who had abnormally high blood fats. They concluded that promoting higher intakes of omega-3 fatty acids in the diet of people with high blood pressure and abnormal blood fats might have substantial benefit in reducing their risk of cognitive decline.

The second study, an offshoot of the ongoing Zutphen Elderly Study, was conducted in three centres in the Netherlands by Boukje and her colleagues. Based on follow-up information from 210 men aged between 70 and 89 years, their test objectives were more specific than the previous two studies in that they focused on the intake of the omega-3 fats DHA and EPA from fish and other foods, which they then compared to patterns of mental decline.

Their results, over five years, were so startling I shall list them:

* Fish eaters had four times less cognitive decline than non-fish eaters.

* The reduction in the risk of mental decline showed a linear dose-effect relationship with the estimated dose of DHA and EPA consumed. This is a very important observation. Indeed, it's the pattern we would look for when testing a new drug, since it points very strongly to a specific beneficial action.

* Those eating the most fish – a daily intake of approximately 380 mg of combined DHA and EPA, which is equivalent to taking a daily fish oil

supplement – were found to have no cognitive decline at all over the five years of study.

This is a very dramatic outcome and we shall look at the reasons why the omega-3s might offer such benefits, but now it is time to look at related studies in the most severe of all types of mental decline – the conditions that come under the umbrella term dementia, and most particularly Alzheimer's disease.

5

Preventing Alzheimer's disease

In *Alice's Adventures in Wonderland*, the Queen of Hearts asks Alice: 'What use is a memory that only works backwards?' The answer, of course, is that memory is precious beyond measure for normal living. Without it we simply cannot function and become lost in a maze of timelessness and indecision.

I witnessed how costly memory loss was about a decade ago when I went to visit my uncle in a long-stay ward, where he had been admitted suffering from Alzheimer's disease. I was all too familiar with the condition, having helped a great many patients and their families come to terms with it. But that did not prepare me for the anguish I felt when I was talking to him. My uncle – let's call him Jim – had been highly intelligent. Moreover, he had always been kind and caring, something I had always treasured. The terrible thing was that I could see and hear that caring intelligence in him even as we spoke, for much of the pride of what he had formerly been was still there, locked away inside. But the destructive effects of his illness had stolen that from him.

The ward was a melancholy place to visit, with kindly nursing staff struggling to look after many patients suffering the indignities of end-stage dementia. During our talks, Jim asked me a single poignant question:

'What am I doing here?'

Patiently, I explained the loss of recent memory that is such a prominent feature of Alzheimer's disease. In his case, memory of distant events, such as the childhood he shared with my father, were a good deal clearer than his memories of a week, or even an hour ago.

His eyes lit up. 'Ah – now I understand!' But minutes later he had forgotten he had even asked me the question.

The experience was so harrowing I have never forgotten it. Witnessing what was happening to him inspired me to write my novel *Between Clouds and the Sea*, in which a young man befriends an old man suffering from depression. I have a profound empathy with people who are looking after loved ones suffering from dementia or depression, and I would like to do what I can to prevent others from suffering this fate.

Jim had dementia; more specifically, Alzheimer's disease, which is the commonest form of dementia. But what does the term dementia mean?

Dementia is a serious and increasingly common disease of the brain in which somebody who was previously normal suffers a progressive loss of cognition and memory. Some memory loss is seen as a natural part of growing older, so much so that you might imagine that dementia is part of the natural ageing process. But this is not so. Dementia, such as we see in Alzheimer's disease, is far from inevitable. As the name of the condition implies it's a *disease*, and that means that, like any other medical affliction, it has causes and the potential of prevention and remedy.

As the Alzheimer's Research Trust, a leading UK research charity for dementia, explains, 'No life blighted by Alzheimer's disease will ever be just a statistic.' Even so the facts and figures of this and other dementias make for sobering reading.

Currently about 800,000 people in the UK are living with dementia. Given the increasing numbers of us living into old age, this number is expected to double in the next twenty years. Some people assume that it is a problem of affluent countries where people live longer than in the developing world, but in fact most people with dementia live in developing countries. Dementia is neither inevitable nor related to standards of living. And that means we need to take a mental step back and look at it clearly and objectively, in all of its aspects.

How does a dementia, such as Alzheimer's disease, first show up?

Often it begins very gradually, so we easily confuse it with the minor memory lapses people have as they grow older. They forget why they came into a room. They may get lost when they go out, perhaps when shopping, and are found wandering. They lose normal reasoning skills like counting change, or make mistakes with everyday activities such as cooking, household chores and personal grooming. Sometimes the frustrations and terror of what is happening show in mood changes or even what appears to be a personality change, with friends and relatives noticing unusual irritability or aggressive behaviour. Please don't panic if you've had minor memory lapses – everybody gets these now and then. The symptoms of depression, for example, often include memory lapses and other features that could easily be mistaken for cognitive decline. It is important that people don't jump the gun or make unwarranted assumptions. But such important caveats aside, a persistent, steady decline in memory may signal the onset of Alzheimer's disease.

Dementia can affect people of any social class or age, but it is more common in older people. It affects 1 in 20 people over the age of 65, and that rises to 1 in 5 people over the age of 80. It really is a major problem, and worry, for society as well as for each and every one of us.

What should you do if you suspect that you, or more likely a relative or friend, is showing signs of dementia? As always, the best thing to do is to consult your GP. Doctors are trained to assess these signs. And if your doctor suspects dementia, there are objective tests, such as brain scans, that can confirm the diagnosis.

So, given that dementias such as Alzheimer's disease are illnesses and not just the process of natural ageing, what causes them?

The answer is there's a number of causes. One common possibility is vascular dementia, which accounts for a little over a quarter of the dementia we see in the UK. This affects men more than women and is brought about by repeated strokes, whether as a result of arteries clogging up or through haemorrhages within the brain, the latter more likely in people who suffer from uncontrolled hypertension. There is a great deal that doctors can do to prevent this type of dementia and help people who have already developed these patterns of disease. Aspirin and the various statin (cholesterol reducing) drugs reduce the risk of blood clots, as does fish oil. And hypertension (high blood pressure) is readily treatable with a wide variety of medications.

Rarer forms of dementia include a condition known as Pick's disease, which can affect people under the age of 65; and there is another disease associated with deposits in the brain known as Lewy bodies. Yet another is the rapidly progressive dementia seen in Creutzfeld Jacob disease – a disastrous affliction which, in the new variant (vCJD), is associated with so-called mad cow disease, caused by eating contaminated beef. I wrote the horrifying story of the origins and implications of mad cow disease in my book *Virus X*. Indeed, if we think about it, any disease that causes a serious interference with brain function will present in much the same way as dementia – slow-growing brain tumours and inflammation, for example. Doctors can readily sort this out and arrive at the correct diagnosis.

What, then, is the cause of Alzheimer's disease, which accounts for almost two-thirds of all the dementia we see in the UK?

The truth is, we don't yet know the cause. What we do know is that it affects more women than men and that it is linked to particular changes in the structure of the brain, with abnormal tangles of nerve cell proteins known as amyloid plaques. There is a lot of inflammation in and around these tangles and it is thought that the inflammation may play an important part in killing nerve cells and thus damaging the surrounding brain structure. Some of the current research is aimed at finding ways of reducing this inflammation. There is a family predisposition in some cases of Alzheimer's disease, linked to a gene that plays a role in handling fats – the APOE gene. However, this gene is not always found, and even if it is, it doesn't mean that the gene is the only causative factor. Indeed, even in the presence of the gene, there is evidence that other factors, including diet, play an important part.

In the longer term, after the disease has been present for some time, the brain shrinks. This can be seen on an MRI scan and more intensive scanning may soon be able to pick up the plaques themselves, offering the possibility of using intensive scanning to assess response to treatments.

Early diagnosis has been pioneered by people such as Andersson at the Caroline Institute, Sweden, who have found ways of testing people who have the disease at the earliest possible stages – even when they are symptom-free. While we might baulk at the idea of being told we are heading for such a terrible disease, an early diagnosis might become crucially important as more effective treatments become available. Some excellent work has also been conducted as part of The Nun Study by colleagues at the University of Kentucky (see 'Other useful sources of information' at the end of this book). And if colleagues at the Institute of Psychiatry, King's College, London, are right, a simple blood test may soon be available to identify people at high risk of developing the disease. This, combined with the ability to diagnose the disease at a very early stage, might be a big step towards better treatment. A similar approach, involving high-risk groups or very early diagnosis, might also offer a more precise means of assessment in dietary prevention trials.

But what, you might ask, can we do to help those people suffering from Alzheimer's disease today?

Unfortunately, although we know a great deal about the disease process in the brain, treatment is far from perfect. Nevertheless, there are some drug therapies in use and others, including gene-based therapies, undergoing research and trials. Relatives and supporters of sufferers can get more information from their GPs and specialist nurses, or from self-help groups such as the Alzheimer's Society, the details of which are given at the end of the book.

I shall pose two questions:

1   Can we reduce the risk of developing Alzheimer's disease by diet?

2   Can we treat people already suffering from Alzheimer's disease through diet?

These questions are important since, if the answer is yes to either one or both, we can do a great deal to help ourselves. I would recommend that you examine the evidence objectively and decide for yourself.

Research in animals suggests that the fish-type omega-3s may have promise in preventing and even treating Alzheimer's disease. For example, a diet rich in DHA reduces or prevents the formation of amyloid tangles in the brains of mice that are prone to develop an Alzheimer pattern of disease. There is even some evidence from these studies that DHA lowers the levels of a chemical that plays a key role in making the tangles. But animal studies, while suggestive, always need to be confirmed in people.

In 1997 a pioneering study was conducted by Kalmijn and colleagues in The Netherlands, which grew out of an ongoing population screening into the causes of diseases and disabilities in older people. Elsewhere, experts had already looked at the impact of malnutrition and the role of saturated fat in dementia. Kalmijn looked more intensively at the different components of the fat in the diet, including total fat, saturated fat, cholesterol and the poly-unsaturated fatty acids including the omega-3s. This carefully formulated study would become the model for similar studies in other countries during the decade that followed.

Their test population, comprising 5,386 volunteers from a suburb of Rotterdam, were aged 55 years and older. People already suffering from dementia were excluded at the beginning and dietary intakes were carefully screened by dieticians. When evidence of dementia was detected during the study, it was confirmed by neurological experts, who conducted MRI imaging of the brain. The study coordinators also screened for other social factors that might possibly be implicated, including age, gender, total calorie intake, cigarette smoking, alcohol consumption, fibre consumption, antioxidant intake and education. They also looked for factors that might be associated with vascular dementia as opposed to Alzheimer's disease – a history of cardiovascular disease and stroke, raised blood fats such as cholesterol, thickening of the arteries in the carotids and high blood pressure.

Fifty-eight of the 5,386 subjects became demented over the period of follow-up, which averaged 2.1 years. Of these, 72 per cent were diagnosed as having Alzheimer's disease, with the others having vascular or other types of dementia. Those who consumed large amounts of saturated fat had an increased risk of developing Alzheimer's disease. Fish consumption was associated with a reduced risk of dementia generally, and especially with a reduced risk of Alzheimer's disease. This conclusion did not change when they allowed for cigarette smoking, alcohol consumption, fibre consumption or antioxidant intake. Nor did it change when they took the levels of blood fats, like cholesterol, or the history of stroke or heart attack, into consideration.

After a discussion of their findings, the Dutch investigators suggested that further population studies should be conducted, and emphasised the need for a longer follow-up period. They also concluded that if their findings were confirmed, this would have important implications for reducing the risk of dementia.

It wasn't long before other studies were being conducted around the world. Two years later, Kyle and colleagues followed up the blood levels of DHA in 1,188 elderly Americans over ten years, to find that Alzheimer's disease was 67 per cent more likely to develop in people with lower DHA levels. That same year in a small trial of DHA treatment of just 20 people suffering from dementia, Terano and colleagues in Japan found that when they divided them into two groups and gave one group DHA supplementation, significant improvement was seen in the dementia scores of the treated group after 3–6 months. But these patients had vascular dementia and not Alzheimer's disease – something we'll consider later. Remember too that the following year, Conquer and her colleagues in Canada analysed the fatty acids in the plasma of patients with Alzheimer's disease, other types of dementia and cognitive impairment, and reported lower blood levels of DHA, total omega-3 fatty acids and also a lower omega-3:omega-6 ratio in Alzheimer's disease and other forms of dementia, as well as in people suffering cognitive decline who were not demented.

In 2002, Barberger-Gateau and colleagues in France followed up 1,674 people aged 68 and over for seven years. Of these, 170 went on to develop dementia, of whom 135 were diagnosed as having Alzheimer's disease. In this large-scale study, consumption of fish or seafood was found to be strongly associated with reduced tendency to dementia. This was particularly true for Alzheimer's disease. They found no association between meat consumption (saturated fat) and risk of dementia. In 2003, Tully and colleagues in Dublin compared the blood levels of EPA and DHA in 168 people suffering from Alzheimer's disease who were still living independently in the community with an equivalent group who did not have the disease. They found the blood levels of both EPA and DHA were significantly lower in the Alzheimer group.

That same year, Morris and her colleagues, at the Rush Institute for Healthy Aging, Chicago, reported in the *Archives of Neurology* on the influence of diet on Alzheimer's disease in 815 volunteers aged 65–94 years. All had normal mental ability at the beginning of their evaluation and were followed up over various periods of time, the average being 3.9 years. During follow-up, 131 developed Alzheimer's disease. In people who consumed fish at least once a week they found that the risk of developing Alzheimer's disease was 60 per cent less than in those who rarely or never ate fish – a similar figure to that obtained by Kyle and colleagues. This protective effect remained true even when they took into account other known risk factors.

It is interesting to note that when they conducted extensive research on the fatty acid content of the fish consumed locally, they found that the strong protective effect was specific for DHA and not EPA – a finding we have come across in other studies, such as the Heude study of cognitive impairment in France. They did admit though that they could not rule out an effect of EPA in the larger doses you would get in fish oil supplements. The vegetable omega-3 alpha-linolenic acid also gave some protection, but this was only found in people carrying the APOE gene.

These results closely paralleled the effects of DHA in animal Alzheimer models. Morris and her colleagues arrived at a conclusion very similar to that of the Rotterdam group. Eating fish, and specifically consuming a regular amount of DHA, might considerably reduce the risk of developing Alzheimer's disease.

Such was the impact of the Chicago study that Dr Friedland, from the Department of Neurology at the School of Medicine, Cleveland, wrote an editorial in the same medical journal with the title 'Fish Consumption and the Risk of Alzheimer Disease: Is it Time to Make Dietary Recommendations?'

We shall return to this question shortly, but we should also consider the fact that not all of the research studies supported these findings. We recall that in 2003 Laurin and her colleagues, reporting from various centres in Canada, disagreed with her Canadian colleagues in finding no link between serum levels of fish type omega-3s and protection from cognitive decline or dementia. More striking still, the Dutch group studying patterns of illness in the elderly in the Rotterdam Study reviewed their data in 2002, and now refuted their earlier findings in a study involving 5,395 people living independently in the community. While they found no link between consumption of omega-3 fatty acids and protection against dementia, they appeared to find a protective effect for consumption of total fat, saturated fat and even cholesterol. These results are puzzling, since they contradict most of the other studies around the world.

In my opinion, occasional conflicting results such as these highlight the difficulties I mentioned earlier in performing mass population studies in which there are so many variables. Yet the question of whether or not the omega-3 fatty acids found in fish oil can help to prevent dementia is a very important one and can only be solved by more high quality, large-scale trials.

In 2006, Schaefer and his colleagues observed 899 American men and women, who had been free of dementia at the start of the study, following their progress for an average of 9.1 years. This study certainly had sufficiency in numbers and a laudable period of follow-up, and was a part of the famous large-scale Framingham Heart Study. All of the test subjects had their plasma levels of fatty acids measured at the beginning of the trial. During follow-up, 99 developed dementia, including 71 cases of Alzheimer's disease. The researchers divided the blood levels of fatty acids into four different quartiles, from high to low, in terms of their DHA content. Those in the highest quartile had roughly 50 per cent less risk of developing dementia in general, and a 40 per cent less risk of developing Alzheimer's disease. I think it significant that here, as in the Zutphen study of the effects of omega-3 fatty acids in cognitive decline, there was a dose-effect relationship, in that the higher the plasma DHA level, the greater the protection. The researchers found no other associations.

When faced with big population studies that show some level of disagreement, doctors look to both the quality of the research and to the majority findings, particularly where the associations are strong and reproduced by different workers in different countries. I believe we have reached that stage.

We might readily think of further studies we would like to see done – for example, in comparing an oily fish diet with fish oil supplements. In time, such studies may well be undertaken. But as long ago as 1990 I suggested the need to conduct large-scale studies comparing fish oil supplements with aspirin in heart attack prevention. I am still waiting. In the meantime, a great many people who took it upon themselves to adopt the message of *The Eskimo Diet* on the evidence then available have reduced their risk of a heart attack. I receive thank-you messages even today from senior medical colleagues as well as lay people.

We've looked at the facts and now we need answers. So let us return to those all-important questions.

* **Can we reduce the risk of cognitive decline by regularly eating oily fish or taking fish oil supplements?**

Given the evidence, coupled with the fact that eating fish or taking a fish oil supplement is so safe and natural, it seems reasonable to say yes.

* **Can we reduce the risk of Alzheimer's disease by regularly eating oily fish or by taking fish oil supplements?**

Once again, it seems reasonable to say yes. We shall look at how to go about this shortly. But first there is another important question.

* **Is taking fish oil a useful treatment for Alzheimer's disease?**

In 2006, Freund-Levi and his colleagues in Stockholm treated people who already had Alzheimer's disease with DHA and EPA. Their study was a controlled medical trial involving 174 patients, who were divided into two groups, one of which was given the omega-3 fatty acids for six months and the other a placebo. Overall the decline of cognition did not differ between the two groups, suggesting that omega-3s are not a cure for developed Alzheimer's disease. However, in a subgroup of 32 milder cases, a definite reduction in mental decline was observed in the omega-3 treated patients.

Although this is only a single, though well-formulated study, it points to the need for additional good quality studies of treatment of early Alzheimer's disease with fish oil or specifically DHA. In 2007 a large-scale study involving 51 centres in the USA was initiated by the Michigan Alzheimer's Disease Research Center. Funded by the National Institutes of Health, it will test the effectiveness of pure DHA in the therapeutic dosage of 2 g daily in people suffering the earliest stages of Alzheimer's disease. We look forward to the results with great interest. In the meantime, given the seriousness of the disease and the relative lack of side-effects from taking fish oil, there would be little to lose in trying fish oil as a treatment in mild cases of Alzheimer's disease.

There is an additional unanswered question:

* **Can we reduce the risk of developing other forms of dementia by regularly eating oily fish or by taking fish oil supplements?**

While Alzheimer's disease is the major cause of dementia, the second biggest cause is disease of the blood vessels to the brain – vascular dementia. A common factor in vascular dementia is blockage of or damage to arteries to the brain, causing the condition known as a stroke. We recall the small-scale investigation in Japan where people suffering from vascular dementia improved when they were given DHA. We might also recall the Beydoun study of cognitive decline in Minneapolis and elsewhere, in which people suffering decline linked to vascular problems appeared to benefit the most. Three major studies have recently been completed in the USA, two encompassing very large numbers of men and women, and a third comprising almost 80,000 nurses aged 34–59. In all of these studies the test populations have been followed for lengthy periods, their fish (and omega-3) consumptions monitored and the incidence of strokes observed. All three studies arrived at a similar conclusion: eating oily fish, or the consumption of fish-type omega-3 fatty acids, reduced the risk of having a stroke. In the nurses group this was significant mainly in those who didn't also take aspirin – a discovery that is not altogether surprising.

Fish oils, and the omega-3s, have more than one action. They not only play a key role in normal brain chemistry, they also reduce the tendency of damaged arteries to develop blood clots – one of the ways in which they reduce heart attacks as well as strokes. This action is similar to that of aspirin and it probably explains why the fish oil takers showed no additional benefit in those taking aspirin in the nurses group.

How does fish oil, and the omega-3s it contains, help reduce the risk of dementia? And how does it help treat milder cases of Alzheimer's disease?

Scientific studies have shown that it does so in a number of different ways, some of which are listed here:

- We already know that fish oil, and DHA specifically, has a vital role in the structural integrity and function of our brains. It is essential for normal brain function. Any dietary deficiency would thus weaken this structural integrity and might increase the risk of malfunction and disease.

- In addition to some gradual loss of nerve cells in the brain as we get older, there are unwanted chemical side-products that impair the function of these nerve cells, with harmful effects on memory and learning capacity. In particular, these lead to an impairment of the ability of nerve cells to transmit signals and messages from one cell to another. This becomes part of a vicious cycle of cholesterol building up in the nerve membranes, making it less fluid, and corrosive chemicals, known as free radicals, further damaging the membrane. This vicious cycle responds to an increase in the omega-3 fatty acids in the diet, in particular DHA.

- EPA and DHA reduce inflammation anywhere in our bodies, which may be a significant way in which they help reduce the risk of developing Alzheimer's disease.

- Within the substance of the brain, DHA cuts down on key chemical pathways that would otherwise lead to the formation of Alzheimer's amyloid tangles.

- EPA and DHA reduce the blood's ability to clot. This contributes to the reduction in risk of vascular dementia.

The omega-3s have other health benefits, which we shall explore shortly, but, given what we now know about the omega-3s, perhaps we shouldn't be too surprised to learn that what helps keep the brain healthy may also keep the mind healthy.

6

Talking about zing

Happiness is the richest prize in life. And while I can't offer you an elixir that will bring it your way, we all know that people who feel at peace with themselves are fun to be with. According to social scientists, they also make more money, have more friends and better jobs and even live longer than their more miserable fellows. So where does happiness come from? It's all down to your inner sense of self-esteem, which in turn is closely related to your mood.

Unfortunately, it would appear that we in Britain are suffering an epidemic of unhappiness, something that's taxing the minds of sociologists. Much research has shown that although we are richer than ever, we are no happier. Moreover, not only does increasing wealth fail to make us happier, but the very means of growing wealthier – all that strife – actually makes a lot of us unhappy.

I can't claim to be a paragon of sense and prudence myself. Like many professionals, I have spent most of my life working long hours and allowing duty to distract me. But it's never too late to slow down a little and think about what can make you happy.

Moreover, I promised you at the very beginning of this book that there was a message that would help to lighten your mood. I promised you a zing thing. And the wonderful message is that your diet really can help you be happy.

If Sarah M. Conklin is right, omega-3 fatty acids may influence areas of the brain that play an important part in our moods and emotions. Dr Conklin, who works in the Department of Psychiatry, University of Pittsburgh, observed that people with lower blood levels of omega-3s were more likely to have a negative outlook than people with higher levels, while those with higher levels felt more at ease with the world and less likely to exhibit the blues. But of course, she and her colleagues didn't content themselves with brain puzzles and teasers, but set out to see whether the volume of grey matter in the brain, especially in areas related to mood, was linked to the amount of omega-3s people consumed.

They measured the amount of omega-3s that 55 healthy adults took in their diets and then used MRI brain scans to calculate the volume of grey matter in certain parts of their brains that are known to play an important part in our moods – the 'zing centres'. What they discovered was that the more omega-3s people ate, the bigger the grey areas associated with their day-to-day moods, and even the regulation of their emotions. Animal studies confirm these findings. Other research has suggested that these areas show a reduced physical volume in people suffering from a negative outlook, which is such a prominent feature of illnesses such as depression.

These studies, which were presented in March 2007 at an international conference, are already triggering further investigation.

But now, perhaps, we should look at the opposite of happiness – the unpleasant illness we know as depression. It appears to be a very common affliction, affecting, according to some estimates, 8 per cent of the population at any given time, and the majority of us at some time in our lives. That's an awful lot of unhappy people. There's an older word for it – melancholia – which appears peculiarly apt. I thought a great deal about the anguish of melancholia while writing my novel *Between Clouds and the Sea*. I went so far as to discuss the illness with a psychiatrist colleague, who had spent a lifetime treating sufferers. He offered me an explanation based on 30 years' experience. In his view a person suffering from depression is going through the mental equivalent of severe and protracted physical pain. The term he used was torture.

How awful, then, to reflect that depression is now recognised as one of the top three causes of disability in the UK, and that the numbers of prescriptions for antidepressants has more than doubled in the last decade. Perhaps most disturbing is the fact that the use of antidepressants and other mind-altering drugs among schoolchildren has more than quadrupled in the same period. In 2006 alone, some 631,000 prescriptions were handed out to children under 16 in the UK, compared with 146,000 in the mid-1990s. Equally shocking are the statistics that show that depression has increased to epidemic levels throughout the Western world. Indeed, according to the World Health Organisation, mental health problems 'are fast becoming the number-one health issue of the 21st century'. There are many very good medical treatments available and anyone who feels that they are suffering from depression, or who believes a friend or relative is suffering, should seek help from their GP. But surely it is time for society to reflect long and hard on what is going on.

My hunch is that the explanation will prove to be complex, but meanwhile, anything that helps prevent such an affliction is clearly welcome. The question I wish to pose now is obvious:

● **Is there any evidence that omega-3 fatty acids might help to alleviate that torture?**

Interest in fish oil as a treatment or prevention of depression surfaced in 1995, when the pioneering US scientist Joseph R. Hibbeln surveyed various countries, including the USA, and suggested that a fall in consumption of the omega-3 fatty acids was directly related to increased rates of depression. For example, rates of depression are 60 times higher in New Zealand than they are in Japan. No doubt there is more than one explanation for this, but Hibbeln thought it might be significant that the Japanese eat four times as much fish as New Zealanders do. In time his observation became the springboard for a number of studies of the effects of marine omega-3s in both the prevention and treatment of depression and the so-called bipolar disorders.

Hibbeln also reported on an international study that looked at seafood consumption in relation to postpartum depression, and he concluded that lower seafood consumption, resulting in less DHA in mother's milk, was associated with higher rates of 'baby blues'. In 2005, with his colleagues, he looked at the effects of adding omega-3s in various dosage regimes to the diet of mothers suffering from postpartum depression. He concluded that the omega-3s resulted in a definite improvement. Moreover, the beneficial effect was noticeable even when they gave sufferers relatively small doses.

A 2003 study published in the *American Journal of Psychiatry* looked at population figures in various countries, this time involving bipolar disorder and seafood consumption, and again they found a strong correlation between bipolar disorder and low consumption of oily fish. In the light of this it seemed relevant that fish consumption has progressively declined in the West over the last two or even three generations. Perhaps, in Hibbeln's opinion, here was at least part of the explanation of why rates of depression had radically increased over the same period. And just this year, a study involving almost 22,000 people in Norway found that people who took cod liver oil regularly had significantly less depression.

Nehmets and his colleagues in Israel looked at what happened when they added fish oil supplements to the maintenance medication in 20 people suffering from severe depression. They concluded that those given the fish oil had 'highly significant benefits' when compared with those given a placebo. This effect was apparent by the third week of treatment.

But not everybody agrees. In a study of 36 depressed patients conducted by Dr Marangell and colleagues at Baylor College of Medicine, Houston, there was no significant effect when they administered pure DHA. However, In 2005, Drs Peet and Stokes reviewed the medical literature on omega-3s and psychiatric disorders and reported that five of six studies into schizophrenia and four of six into depression found therapeutic benefit from treatment with omega-3s. They rightly concluded that larger prospective studies are needed.

It's fair to say that it is too early to make confident predictions. However, there would appear to be little to lose if people who are suffering from depression were to eat more oily fish or take a modest omega-3 supplement daily (provided they are not in the small minority who are allergic to fish, or who otherwise need to be cautious about taking fish oil).

Preventing heart attacks and treating autoimmune conditions

In 2007, some 17 years after *The Eskimo Diet* came out, the UK National Institute for Health and Clinical Excellence (NICE) recommended that patients who had suffered a heart attack in the previous three months, and who declined or were unable to eat two or more portions of oily fish a week, should be given fish oil supplements to reduce the risk of further heart attacks. Similar advice had already been given in the diet and lifestyle recommendations of the American Heart Association. This reflected the findings of one of the biggest prospective studies ever conducted, involving 11,323 patients who had already had a heart attack, and reported in 2002 by a multi-centre group of Italian researchers. They concluded that there was a significant reduction in mortality in those given omega-3 supplements.

It is outside the remit of this book to review the extensive evidence for fish oil in heart attack prevention, but it is reasonable to say that the evidence since 1990 has amply confirmed our advice at that time.

I have suffered from arthritis for 17 years, during which time I have taken a dessertspoon of cod liver oil daily to help control my symptoms. Although I don't claim this has cured the condition, it has enabled me to avoid taking anti-inflammatory drugs for most of the time. This will hardly come as a surprise to many fellow sufferers, since people have known about the benefits of cod liver oil for centuries. As long ago as 1782 a doctor named Thomas Percival was using cod liver oil to treat the symptoms of arthritis, while even earlier another doctor, Samuel Kay, working at the Manchester Infirmary, extolled it in the treatment of many different bony disorders.

Broadly speaking, there are two categories of arthritis: inflammatory arthritis, where the membranes around the joints become inflamed because of an immune reaction; and osteoarthritis, where the inflammation is the result of wear and tear within the joint. Osteoarthritis tends to affect one or just a few joints – knees and hips, or the little but much used joints of the thumbs and fingers. Inflammatory arthritis is usually widespread and often symmetrical, for example in rheumatoid arthritis and, to a lesser degree, in lupus.

Until recently – and in spite of the fact that people with osteoarthritis swore they benefited – doctors believed that fish oil, with its property of damping down inflammation, mainly benefited the inflammatory forms of arthritis rather than osteoarthritis. But work by Professor Bruce Caterson and colleagues at Cardiff University looked at how omega-3s actually help inflamed joints. Recognising that arthritis, whatever its origin, involves inflammation and ultimately destruction of the cartilage surrounding the joints, they looked at what happened when they added omega-3s to the cartilage cells in conditions that mimicked inflammation. The products of certain 'inflammatory genes' are carried into the cartilage where they give rise to pain and inflammation. The Cardiff scientists found that the omega-3s block the effects of these inflammatory genes. In their summing up they wrote: 'These findings ... advocate a beneficial role for dietary fish oil supplementation in alleviation of several of the physiological parameters that cause and propagate arthritic disease.'

Given their anti-inflammation effects, it will come as no surprise that omega-3s have been assessed as a treatment in a wide variety of autoimmune diseases, including rheumatoid arthritis, lupus, psoriasis, multiple sclerosis and the bowel diseases, ulcerative colitis and Crohn's disease. The clearest benefit has been in rheumatoid arthritis and lupus, whereas in other conditions such as asthma and the inflammatory bowel diseases, the benefit was harder to demonstrate.

There is also some – albeit early – evidence that omega-3s may play a role in reducing the risk of developing some kinds of cancer. But in my view, we need a good deal more information before it is possible to make predictions, or recommendations.

How, we might reasonably ask, could such simple natural substance as fish oil be capable of offering us this rainbow of benefit?

The answer, as so often with important scientific truths, is complex. The most important thing to grasp is that the fish oil omega-3s DHA and EPA are essential fatty acids. This means that we need them for normal health, just like vitamins. They play an important role in our body chemistry and defences – so part of what we are witnessing in these studies is not the application of a drug to treat a disease, but the correction of a dietary deficiency of a vitamin-like ingredient that is a normal requirement for human health.

However, several of the big studies also suggest a more therapeutic role in conditions such as arthritis, lupus, cognitive decline and mild Alzheimer's disease in taking a daily supplement as opposed to eating oily fish one or two days a week. We are only beginning to understand some of the complex actions of fish oil in these conditions, whether it results in a reduction of inflammation, a switching off of damaging gene expression or more subtle interaction with the body's internal chemistry, such as brain cell-to-cell communication.

8

The all-important ratio of omega-3s to omega-6s

It should be obvious by now that a healthy diet should be as close to natural as possible. Much less obvious is how to go about correcting the unhealthy eating patterns that so many of us have fallen into. Of course, there is more to healthy eating than just increasing the amount of oily fish we eat or the omega-3s we add as supplements, and I shall explain this in the next chapters. But for the moment let us focus on the most complex of these issues – getting the right balance of fats in your diet. This subject could become unnecessarily confusing so I shall explain it in four simple steps.

1   The total amount of fat recommended for a healthy adult diet is 80 g (roughly 2½–3 oz) a day.

2   Of this at least 30 g (1 oz) should be unsaturated fat. This should include olive oil (for the monounsaturated oleic acid) and the various polyunsaturated fatty acids, including omega-6s and omega-3s.

3   Of this unsaturated fat, the ideal ratio of omega-6 to omega-3 is 4:1. This ratio, which has never been published in any popular literature before, is based on research by Yehuda and his colleagues in Israel and

elsewhere, and it suggests that an adult diet should contain 6 g of omega-3s a day. This is far more than the quantity of EPA and DHA recommended above. But remember that the omega-3s in this sense includes those of common vegetable origins, such as alpha-linolenic acid, or ALA.

4   Of the 6 g of omega-3s, you will get what you need of DHA and EPA from eating a minimum of two oily fish meals a week, or by taking an omega-3 supplement that gives you a minimum of 400 mg combined EPA and DHA a day. In fact, the recommended dosage varies, depending on whether or not you already have a relevant medical condition, or might be at high risk of developing a relevant medical condition. I shall go on to explain this further.

Eating a fish meal at least twice a week is not only attractive and palatable, it has the advantage of replacing red meat as a main dish on the day you eat it, so reducing your intake of saturated fat into the bargain. The minimum amount recommended is equivalent to 200 g (7 oz) of mackerel a week or 325 g (11 oz) of wild salmon. If, however, you are suffering from a condition such as arthritis that might be alleviated by fish oil, you might consider taking a daily supplement of fish oil as part of your diet. On pragmatic grounds, people who for one reason or another are unable or unwilling to eat oily fish – and surveys in the UK suggest that as many as seven out of ten people feel that way – should consider taking a daily supplement of fish oil as a normal and regular part of their diet. The same advice applies to those of you who worry that you are at increased risk of cognitive decline, dementia or suffering a heart attack, with the precautions and contraindications already mentioned, for example in people who have a bleeding tendency or who are taking aspirin or warfarin.

This is exactly what I have been doing for the last 17 years – and shall continue to do for the rest of my life.

Some people might disagree that fish oil supplements are natural, but we need to consider what's really natural these days when the marine environments can be polluted with toxic wastes, such as mercury, and much of the fish and shellfish we eat are not wild at all but farm-reared, which sometimes involves the stock being fed artificial diets. I don't wish to exaggerate the fear of pollutants in fish. It would be a sad day indeed if people were frightened of eating such a healthy food. But I do advocate prudence. Fish oil purchased from a reputable manufacturer should have been screened for toxins. Moreover, it should also contain a reliable amount of DHA and EPA, so you can get your daily quota right. With farmed fish and shellfish this is a little more problematic. It seems reasonable to ask that fish and shellfish farms should subject their stocks to regular and independent checks for pollutants and omega-3 content. What better advertisement could they give for their product than to be able to state with confidence that it is wholesome and contains the 'wild' level of the health-giving omega-3s!

We are about to examine fish for omega-3 content and how to incorporate oily fish into our diet. Meanwhile people may have questions about fish oil and omega-3 supplements and I shall try to answer some of these.

✸ Whom do I recommend the brain food diet to?

The answer is, of course, everyone, other than the tiny minority who are allergic to fish or shellfish, or who, for some medical reason, are unable to take fish oil. It must be obvious that the omega-3 fatty acids are very important in many different aspects of our body chemistry. They are essential to health in the strict medical sense – and every bit as important as vitamins. That need begins in the womb and continues right to the very end of our lives.

❋ Where do the omega-3s in fish come from?

Fish can no more manufacture the essential EPA and DHA fatty acids than we can. They obtain theirs from plankton and algae. This is why we need to be a little cautious about fish that have been bred in farms – it's all a question of whether they feed naturally or not. If they are fed soybean or other plant seeds or grains, or worse still, saturated fat, they may be relatively poor suppliers of EPA and DHA. As a general rule, fish taken from the sea are the best providers.

The way we cook fish can also affect the oily content. Frying removes some of the oils. Grilling, baking or poaching offer the best means of guaranteeing goodness. You should, however, avoid boiling since that also removes the oils from the flesh. This is a problem with some brands of tinned tuna, which are boiled so dry they have a much reduced omega-3 content, before being reconstituted in vegetable oil, high in omega-6s. Better to buy tuna canned in brine since this reduces the omega-6:omega-3 ratio.

❋ Which fish oil or omega-3 supplement should I take?

Pregnant and breast-feeding mums are advised to eat oily fish, but, as the Food Standards Agency cautions, they should limit this to two portions of fish a week (a portion is about 150 g (5 oz)). The caution is necessary because of the pollution of rivers, lakes and oceans with toxins such as mercury, pesticides, PCBs and dioxins. This danger is greater in fish caught in lakes than fish caught in the oceans. Moreover, mercury is more of a problem with fish that live long, and thus have more time to accumulate it, such as shark, swordfish and larger species of tuna. The tip, then, is to choose small fish – sardines, herrings or mackerel. If a pregnant woman hates fish, she should seek the advice of her GP, obstetric nurse or obstetrician. With cod liver oil there is some concern about overdosing with vitamin A during pregnancy. Quality cod liver oil contains the RDA (Recommended Daily Allowance) of vitamin A. Some manufacturers have taken out the vitamin A, but you still receive vitamin D and the omega-3s. A small dose of pure fish oil, which contains little or no vitamin A, might offer a solution – but always consult a GP, obstetric nurse or obstetrician before taking any health supplement.

Children should also eat oily fish. But if they can't, or won't, an omega-3 supplement such as *Haliborange* should be considered.

As for adults, there are a number of fish oils on the market and even more varieties of omega-3 supplements, so it's hardly surprising people get confused. When it comes to making a choice, my answer is simple. Choose a fish oil, or cod liver oil, that comes from a reliable manufacturer. What do I mean by reliable? I would choose a manufacturer that has provided oils for medical and scientific trials. That way you know they employ knowledgeable scientists and their oils will have been tested. This is important since reputable manufacturers will take measures to exclude pollutants, such as mercury, from their products and the doses of omega-3s will be safe and reliable. If you are uncertain about your manufacturer, why not write to them and ask if their oil has been supplied for medical studies. You might also ask about the exclusion of pollutants and the reliability of the omega-3 content.

☀ Which oil do I take?

I take *Seven Seas High Strength Cod Liver Oil*. I chose it for two reasons: the doses of EPA and DHA are right for treating arthritis, and I have a family history of heart attacks. There's the additional and important bonus that it comes from a reputable manufacturer and so I know that it is screened and purified to avoid pollutants and is carefully monitored to provide a reliable quantity of omega-3s. You will already be getting an important message, that the recommended doses for arthritis – 800 mg of combined EPA and DHA a day – is different from the recommended dose for preventing cognitive decline, which is half this amount.

☀ Exactly what dose of omega-3 should I aim for?

Once you have chosen the oil you wish to buy, work out your needs from how much omega-3 fatty acids it contains. For heart attack prevention, as with arthritis, the recommended dose is approximately 800 mg of omega-3s a day. You can calculate this by adding the amount of EPA and DHA in the oil or concentrate. Usually, it will be between a teaspoon and a dessertspoon – the typical chemist's 5 ml spoon is usually about right. The recommended dose for prevention of Alzheimer's disease or prevention of cognitive decline is roughly 400 mg per day. Capsules are a good alternative for people who don't like the taste of oil.

✸ Will I experience any side-effects?

Millions of people in the UK take fish oils every day. Indeed, for the vast majority of the population, fish oil supplementation in these small doses is eminently safe. This is because it is not a medication in the usual sense but the natural oil you would eat in a small portion of oily fish.

✸ Should anyone avoid taking fish oil supplements?

A small minority need to be cautious about taking fish oil. It is essential that people who are taking anticoagulant drugs, such as warfarin or aspirin, should avoid taking fish oil supplements because fish oil slows blood clotting – which is one of the reasons why it helps to reduce the risk of a heart attack. We want to avoid fish oil and the anticoagulant drugs from adding to each other. For the same reason, people who have suffered from a cerebral haemorrhage or a bleeding disorder of any kind should avoid taking fish oil.

Some doctors believe that people with diabetes also need to be cautious because fish oil reduces harmful cholesterol and triglycerides in the blood. While these effects are highly desirable in reducing the risk of a heart attack, people with diabetes are said to show a different response in their blood fats. But this needs to be balanced against the fact that people with diabetes have an increased risk of arterial disease, and a number of studies, including a recent investigation by Hu and his colleagues at Harvard, involving 5,103 nurses with diabetes, showed a marked reduction in death rate from heart attacks in those who ate oily fish. They also noted that fish oil supplementation did not impair blood sugar control. Indeed, they recommended that oily fish should be considered an integral part of the healthy diet of people suffering from diabetes. The simple answer, as always, is that if you have any worries about taking fish oil, consult your GP.

● What's the difference between fish oil and cod liver oil?

Pure fish oil is extracted from fish flesh (the meaty muscle), whereas cod liver oil, as the name suggests, is extracted from liver. This means that, unlike pure fish oil, cod liver oil contains vitamin D and vitamin A as well as the omega-3 fatty acids DHA and EPA. Pure fish oil is also a little more palatable since it has less fishy taste. Some fruit flavoured oils are now available and children like these.

● What if, for family or personal reasons I believe that I am at relatively high risk of cognitive decline or developing Alzheimer's disease – should I take a higher dose?

You will recall that there appeared to be a dose response in some of the big population studies, which would suggest that people at higher risk might benefit from taking a higher dose. I see no reason why somebody at increased risk of Alzheimer's disease, or who is already experiencing early signs of either condition, shouldn't take up to 800 mg of the omega-3s, which will also benefit the heart and whole body health. However, 400 mg daily is generally recommended for maintaining memory and mental agility in people concerned about cognitive decline.

9

Planning your diet

Healthy eating for the brain and mind – that's what this book is all about. And if we can combine healthy eating with happy eating, so much the better! It's clear from many of the big population studies that the experts are telling us that healthy eating isn't about taking care of ourselves with a single dietary ingredient. Again and again, they highlight the importance of getting the balance right between different ingredients, and most important of all between different types of fats. If all you needed to do was add more omega-3s to your diet, I wouldn't need to write a whole book. I could say it in a sentence. But that would only give you part – albeit a key part – of the story. As we have seen, critical among these essential balances is the ratio of unsaturated to saturated fats, and among the unsaturated fats the ratio of omega-3s to omega-6s.

Some time ago a 40-year-old woman came to my clinic complaining of painful bones. An X-ray revealed hairline cracks in some of her major bones, and I diagnosed vitamin D deficiency. When the hospital dieticians investigated her diet, she was found to be on a weight-loss diet that was grossly deficient in fat. We corrected her vitamin D deficiency and put her on a healthier diet, and her condition recovered to normal.

How did this unfortunate condition come about?

For a generation or more, people have assumed that all fat is bad for us. As a result some people put themselves on fad diets, which recommend that a particular item, such as fat, is drastically reduced. In part, this anti-fat bias arose from the demonising of cholesterol as a major contributor to heart attack, when in fact cholesterol taken in moderation is a normal component of our body chemistry. This patient believed she had to cut out as much fat as possible from her diet. The result? A very serious dietary deficiency.

As always, it's a question of getting the balance right.

You may say, 'Well, everyone knows that healthy eating is based on a balanced diet!' You're wrong. Just like this lady, a lot of people don't understand what the word 'balanced' really means. And who could blame them when they're being bombarded by conflicting advice, much of it from uninformed sources. Getting that very desirable balance is not as easy as people assume. How can we balance the various types of fats when we're shopping at the supermarket, or thinking ahead to the meals we give our families day to day and week to week?

It's all a little more complex than merely adding omega-3s to the diet. But don't worry. We shall sort this out in these next three chapters, and all in the simplest and most practical of ways.

Let me say at the very outset that the best advice is to avoid fad diets altogether. We all need a reasonable amount of fat in our diets since without it we become ill through deficiency of the essential fatty acids as well as the fat-soluble vitamins D, E, K and A. Moreover, there's nothing wrong with carbohydrates, another natural food that has frequently been demonised, yet which is an excellent source of readily available energy and often linked to key nutrients like vitamin B1 and folic acid. Most dieticians would recommend that, wherever possible, we take our carbohydrates in complex form. I shall show you how to do this below.

What I suggest, then, is no more than a sensible approach, based on an enjoyable and nutritious balance of wholesome ingredients. It shouldn't be difficult to take on board, and I hope you'll find it pleasurable.

The most common deficiency in the UK is the fish-derived omega-3s, since many of us no longer eat enough oily fish. Indeed, modern food production and processing, including baked goods and rearing of meat and dairy animals on grain rather than grass, tends to overload the balance even further towards omega-6 fatty acids. Clearly, we need not only to put the omega-3s back where they belong, as a core ingredient of our everyday diet, but also to balance this against an excessive intake of omega-6s. What better way to do this than to reduce our reliance on convenience foods and do more proper cooking, allowing us to take charge of those important ingredients ourselves! It's time that society realised the value and pleasure of good, wholesome home cooking.

There is also some evidence that antioxidants, such as vitamins C and E, may have a protective role in cognition and dementia. Vitamin C, or ascorbic acid, is a water-soluble vitamin found in many foods, including vegetables, fruits and meats, so deficiency is unlikely in a balanced diet. Vitamin E is a fat-soluble vitamin found in vegetable fats and oils, and also in cod liver oil. About a quarter of the average daily intake comes from margarines and similar spreads. Again, it is so widely distributed in natural foods that deficiency is unlikely in a balanced diet. There is growing evidence that beta-carotene, a precursor of vitamin A, may help to keep our arteries healthy while also protecting our brain against anti-oxidant damage. Dark green leaves are an excellent source.

Beta-carotene (the name comes from carrot) is just one example of a group of healthy ingredients responsible for the bright colours of fruits and vegetables, which, in the nutritional jargon, are grouped together as carotenoids. Spinach, kiwis, kale and egg-yolk are all excellent sources of another carotenoid, lutein, which reduces the risk of macular degeneration of the retina – a disease that is often, though not always, associated with ageing. Lutein and lycopene, the pigment that makes tomatoes red, also protect our skin from the damaging effects of UV light.

Vitamin A, which is closely related to some of these compounds, is also found in a wide variety of foods, including cod liver oil.

Here, then, is a working plan for healthy and happy eating that aims to take all of these considerations on board.

1 Eat oily fish at least twice a week or balance your diet with a daily supplement of fish oil. Choose small fish, if possible – mackerel, herrings, sardines and pilchards. And remember that shellfish are often excellent providers of omega-3s.

2 Eat roughly 80 g (2½–3 oz) of fat a day, keeping the amount of saturated fat relatively low by replacing it with polyunsaturates and monounsaturates.

● **TIP: Saturated fats are hard at room temperatures whereas unsaturated fats are liquid.**

3   Eat less refined sugar, replacing it with complex
    carbohydrates, such as bread, pasta, high-fibre
    breakfast cereals, and boiled, baked or mashed
    potatoes. Refined sugars, including those used to
    sweeten processed foods, raise your blood sugar rapidly
    and cause a surge in insulin requirements, which
    increases the risk of hypertension, diabetes, heart
    disease and stroke. Bread is not only an excellent
    source of complex carbohydrate, it is also fortified with
    iron, calcium and the B vitamins thiamine and niacin,
    and the milled flour used to make bread in the UK
    may soon be fortified (as it is in the USA and Canada)
    with folic acid, to prevent neural tube abnormalities in
    the foetus.

4   Keep your intake of salt down. Too much puts you at
    risk of hypertension, vascular stroke and dementia.
    The Food Standards Agency recommend no more than
    6 g of salt a day for an adult, but considerably less for
    children and less again in infancy. Much tighter
    controls are necessary for people with kidney disease. I
    would recommend that parents familiarise themselves
    with the Food Standards Agency website – see the
    on-line address at the end of this book.

● **TIP: Try taking pepper rather than salt as a condiment. You might get to like it.**

5   Fibre, or 'roughage', is the skeletal structure of many
    plants, such as wheat, oats and corn, and many

vegetables and fruit. Fibre keeps down cholesterol, which increases the risk of vascular dementia and also damages nerve cell membranes. It also helps prevent constipation and irritable bowel disease and may help to prevent diabetes, heart attacks and colon cancer. Excellent sources of fibre include fruit and vegetables and high-fibre cereals, such as bran flakes, Weetabix and All-bran. Sweeten your breakfast cereal with raisins or sultanas (reduces the intake of refined sugars) and a sprinkling of fresh walnuts (reduces cholesterol). Use skimmed or semi-skimmed milk to reduce saturated fat.

6 Make sure you have a good intake of vitamins by eating fruit and vegetables. This reduces antioxidant damage to the brain and may help reduce the risk of cognitive decline and dementia. The recommendation is that we eat five portions of vegetables and fruit a day. If this seems a tall order, remember a glass of fruit juice or tomato juice counts as one portion – but beware of added salt in tomato juice. Otherwise a portion amounts to a whole fruit, such as an apple, pear, orange or banana, or a whole vegetable such as a pepper, onion, two average size tomatoes, or half an avocado. At dinner, three tablespoons of vegetables, such as peas or carrots, amounts to a portion. Frozen fruit or vegetables retain all of their valuable nutrients. Salads are excellent sources of fibre and vitamins, as are steamed vegetables. To get all the important carotenoids, try to mix the colours: dark green, light green, purple, orange and red.

7   Enjoy a drink, but go easy on the alcohol, which is detrimental to the brain and when taken to excess causes serious liver, brain and peripheral nerve damage. Red wine is beneficial to the heart, but only in modest quantities. When possible try to take wine with a meal rather than on its own, when rapid absorption leads to high blood levels.

8   Above all aim for a diet that it is varied and enjoyable. The guiding principle is to increase, not decrease, the joy of good and healthy eating.

In the next chapter, I have included sample recipes which will not only help to conserve your brain health and function but will also give you a rough guide on how to develop these ideas for yourself.

❋ Which are the oily fish?

The following table gives you the omega-3 content for specific fish – but bear in mind that these are relatively crude figures and apply to fish caught in the wild. Amounts of omega-3s will vary according to where the fish was caught and even the time of year.

Fish contain very different amounts of the protective omega-3s. For instance, the edible portions of cod, haddock and plaice, the British favourites, are all modest providers. If you enjoy these fish and you don't like oily fish, I would suggest you continue to eat the fish you like – preferably not battered and fried – and take the omega-3s as supplements.

The table (modified from an authoritative report by Hepburn, Exler and Weihrauch, 'Provisional tables on the content of omega-3 fatty acids and other fat components of selected sea-foods', *Journal of the American Dietetic Association*) lists the beneficial oils in most of commonly purchased fish, together with many less commonly purchased. The fish are grouped in three sections: most beneficial, moderately beneficial and least beneficial.

Most readers will be familiar with purchasing and cooking fish. Those of you who aren't might start with the more common, highly beneficial varieties, and then, with experience, experiment a little – ask your fishmonger or market trader about some of the less common types of fish.

The table assumes fresh fish and uncooked weight. The approximate omega-3 content is expressed as milligrams of fatty acid per 100 g (3.5 oz) helping.

High fatty fish (most beneficial)

mackerel 2,200	bluefish 1,200
spiny dogfish 2,000	mullet (unspecified) 1,100
herring (sardines) 1,700	Greenland halibut 900
pilchards 1,700	striped bass 800
salmon 1,400	freshwater bass 300
bluefin tuna 1,600	striped mullet 600
lake trout 1,600	oyster 600
rainbow trout 600	carp 600
trout (Arctic char) 600	squid (short-finned) 600
trout (brook) 600	squid (Atlantic) 400
Atlantic sturgeon 400	squid (unspecified) 300
common sturgeon 400	skipjack tuna 500
anchovy 1,400	other (unspecified) tuna 500
sprat 1,300	

Medium fatty fish (moderately beneficial)

hake (unspecified) 500	pollock 500
Pacific hake 400	sea-bass 400
Atlantic hake 100	shrimp 400
blue mussel 500	crab 400
periwinkle 500	white perch 400
shark 500	yellow perch 300
catfish (brown bullhead) 500	ocean perch 200
catfish (channel) 300	

Poor fatty fish (least beneficial)

pike (wall-eye) 300	scallop 200
pike (northern) 100	flounder 200
clam 300	lobster 200
Atlantic cod 300	eel 200
Pacific cod 200	abalone 100
plaice (European) 200	haddock 100

Try to extend your range of dishes and tastes, and remember that what seems strange and new may need several attempts with different recipes before you learn to appreciate its attractiveness and flavour. In the next chapter you'll find some fish recipes to show you how easily this can be achieved. I hope you enjoy them.

10

Brain food recipes

Many nutritionists recommend that we adopt aspects of the so-called Mediterranean diet, which is rich in unsaturated fatty acids. As Solfrizzi and his colleagues have shown in a study of 278 Italians, aged between 65 and 84 years, a diet high in monounsaturated fatty acids, such as you find in olive oil, also appears to give some protection against age-related cognitive decline. These folks certainly enjoyed a very low incidence of age-related cognitive decline. But in extolling the virtues of olive oil, we shouldn't ignore the fact that people in Greece, Italy and Spain eat far more oily fish than we do in the UK – indeed fish is the Spanish national dish.

So, we shall begin this recipe section with a tip on preparing a suitable Mediterranean sauce that goes well with many fish recipes. I'm grateful to a former colleague from the Basque Country who gave me this simple and delicious recipe.

Mullet with Basque sauce

Serves 2

Basque sauces are usually prepared as an integral part of cooking the fish. This has many advantages – for example, it avoids the saturated butter fat that is often included in white sauces, as well as flour to thicken the sauce. What's more, the vegetables offer one of the five healthy portions to your diet.

30 ml (2 tablespoons) of olive oil
1 small onion, skinned and sliced
1 clove garlic, skinned and crushed
½ green pepper, deseeded and sliced
150 ml (¼ pint) white wine, preferably *Vinho Verde*
450 g (1 lb) mullet
salt and freshly ground pepper
chopped fresh parsley

TIP: Olive oil is fine in Mediterranean cooking and sauces, but it may be too strong in traditional British cooking.

To enjoy this dish the true Basque way, cook the fish in an earthenware dish.

Put the oil, onion, garlic and green pepper in a saucepan and cook slowly over a low heat for about 10 minutes, stirring occasionally. Add 30 ml (2 tablespoons) wine and cook for another 3 minutes.

Place the fish in an earthenware dish, add the freshly cooked sauce and pour in the remainder of the wine. Add a little salt and pepper and sprinkle with parsley. Cook in a preheated oven at 180 °C (350 °F, mark 4) for 15 minutes.

Remove from the oven, shake the dish gently, baste with sauce and cook for a further 10 minutes.

Baked salmon steaks

Serves 4
600 g (1¼ lb) salmon
30 ml (2 tablespoons) sunflower seed oil
salt and freshly ground black pepper
Basque sauce

Pre-heat the oven to 240°C (500°F, mark 9).

Place the fish on a pre-heated, oiled baking tin. Add sunflower seed oil and sprinkle with salt and ground pepper. Bake until the fish flakes easily. Serve with Basque sauce, new potatoes and vegetables.

TIP: A lot of the salt we take is added to food, whether in the processing or during cooking. Be relatively frugal with salt in cooking.

Savoury sea bass

Serves 4
4 sea bass fillets
2 tablespoons chopped parsley and chives
2 tablespoons sunflower oil
15 ml (1 tablespoon) lemon juice
salt and pepper to taste
lemon slices

Season the fish. Place in a grill pan and pour the oil over the fish. Grill under moderate heat for about 12–15 minutes (depending on thickness). Turn once. Transfer the fish to a preheated serving dish. Pour the contents of the grill pan into a saucepan adding the lemon juice and herbs. Heat but do not boil, with continuous stirring, and pour over the fish.

Serve with new potatoes and green vegetables.

Pickled herrings

Serves 4

4 herrings, cleaned, heads, tails and backbone removed
sliced onion rings
150 ml (¼ pint) vinegar
50 ml (3 tablespoons) of water
a little plain flour
salt and pepper

Preheat the oven to 180 °C (35 °F, mark 4).

Clean the fillets by rubbing with a little salt and remove fins. Coat in seasoned flour, roll up and place in ovenproof dish. Top with onion rings. Pour over the vinegar and water mixture. Cover and bake in a preheated oven for approximately 35 minutes removing lid about 10 minutes before end of cooking time to brown slightly.

Serve with salad and wholemeal bread.

Seafood paella

Serves 4

300 g (10 oz) fish of your choice (white fish is fine since the shellfish contain additional omega-3s)
225 g (8 oz) raw prawns
12 mussels

200 g (7oz) long grained rice
1 medium onion, finely chopped
2 cloves garlic
30 ml (2 tablespoons) olive oil
1 large red pepper, chopped
1 large green pepper, chopped
a few strands of saffron
180 g (6oz) frozen peas, defrosted
200 ml (⅓ pint) hot fish or vegetable stock
¼ teaspoon paprika
chopped parsley
lemon wedges to serve

Scrub and de-beard the mussels. Place in a large pan with a cupful (200 ml) of water, cover and cook for 5 minutes, shaking the pan from time to time. Discard any mussels that do not open.

Peel and de-vein the prawns, leaving the tails intact. Cut the fish into bite-sized cubes.

Heat the olive oil in a large, deep frying pan. Add the onion and fry for about 2 minutes. Add the garlic and peppers and stir well. Add the rice, stirring well to coat in the oil, then add the saffron and paprika. Pour in the stock and stir thoroughly. Bring to the boil and simmer for about 7 minutes, making sure the rice doesn't stick to the pan. Add the fish, mussels and prawns and continue cooking until the rice is tender and the fish is cooked.

Add a splash of white wine or more stock if the mixture becomes too dry. Sprinkle with chopped parsley and serve with lemon wedges.

Smoked mackerel and apple cocktail

Serves 4
2 smoked mackerel fillets, skinned
2 dessert apples, diced
15 ml (1 tablespoon) lemon juice
5 cm (2 in) piece of cucumber, diced
2 stalks celery, diced
30 ml (2 tablespoons) mayonnaise
45 ml (3 tablespoons) natural yoghurt
5 ml (1 teaspoon) French mustard
grated rind of one orange
salt and pepper

Flake the fish fillets. Toss the apple in lemon juice in a large bowl, then add the mackerel and other ingredients. Stir well and season. Divide between four shallow dishes and serve with wholemeal bread.

Mackerel baked potatoes

Serves 2
225 g (8 oz) smoked mackerel fillets, skinned
15 ml (1 tablespoon) horseradish sauce (optional)
ground black pepper
2 × 225 g (8 oz) potatoes
skimmed milk
30 g (1 oz) cheese (low to medium fat), grated

Bake potatoes until cooked. Flake the mackerel into a bowl, mix in the horseradish sauce (if using) and season with pepper. Slice open potatoes and scoop out the contents, retaining the skins for further use. Mix potato with fish mixture, then put back into the potato, sprinkle with cheese and place under a medium grill until cheese has melted.

Serve hot with a mixed salad.

Mackerel fillets with mushrooms

Serves 4
4 mackerel fillets
180 g (6 oz) mushrooms, quartered
30 ml (2 tablespoons) lemon juice
salt and freshly ground black pepper

Preheat the oven to 375 °C (190 °F, mark 5).

Place the mackerel fillets, skin side down, in an oven-proof dish. Sprinkle with the mushrooms, lemon juice and seasoning. Cover and bake in a preheated over for 25–30 minutes.

Serve with salad.

Kipper soup

Serves 6
450 g (1 lb) kipper fillets
2 x 400g (14 oz) cans tomatoes
2 cloves garlic
30 ml (2 tablespoons) tomato purée
200 ml (⅓ pint) skimmed milk
freshly ground black pepper
1 teaspoon sugar
a little natural yoghurt to serve (optional)
crusty wholemeal bread, warmed briefly in the oven

Chop kippers into small pieces. Blend the tomatoes and

garlic to a soupy consistency. Add the kippers, sugar and tomato puree, and blend again. Transfer to a saucepan, stir in the milk and season with pepper before bringing to the boil. Lower heat and simmer for 5 minutes. Serve with a splash of yoghurt (if desired) and hot crusty wholemeal bread.

Seafood tagliatelle

Serves 4–5

15 ml (1 tablespoon) olive oil
1 small onion, finely chopped
15 g (1 rounded tablespoon) plain flour
300 ml (½ pint) semi-skimmed milk
150 ml (¼ pint) water
salt and freshly ground black pepper
120–150 g (4–6 oz) button mushrooms, sliced
450 g (1 lb) haddock fillet, skinned and cubed
60–120 g (2–4 oz) peeled prawns
225 g (8 oz) green tagliatelle
1 tablespoon corn flour (optional, for a thicker sauce)

Fry the chopped onion in the olive oil until softened but not brown. Add the flour and cook for one minute over a medium heat. Remove from heat and gradually stir in the milk. Return to the heat and cook, stirring constantly until sauce is smooth and thickened. Reduce heat and stir in the water. Season and stir in mushrooms and haddock

Simmer gently, stirring occasionally, for about 5 minutes until haddock is cooked. Stir in prawns and continue cooking for 1–2 minutes until prawns are hot.

If a thicker sauce is required, mix the corn flour with a

little water and incorporate into the sauce before adding the haddock.

Cook the pasta in boiling salted water for about 8 minutes or according to instructions on the packet. Drain and serve with the fish sauce.

Smoked mackerel pâté

Serves 4
180 g (6 oz) smoked mackerel fillets
juice of ½ lemon
75 g (2½ oz) low-fat cheese
5 ml (l teaspoon) horseradish sauce
pepper to taste

Skin, flake and bone the mackerel, squeeze lemon into it, add other ingredients and mix thoroughly. Put mixture in a serving bowl and decorate with thinly sliced lemon. Chill for several hours before serving.

Salmon or trout can also be used, but more seasoning is required.

Salmon pâté

Serves 6
225 g (8 oz) cooked salmon
15 ml (l tablespoon) tomato purée
15 g (½ oz) butter
15 g (½ oz) plain flour
300 ml (½ pint) semi-skimmed milk
salt and pepper
1 sachet of gelatine, dissolved in 3 tablespoonfuls of warm
    water

juice of half a lemon
small carton of natural yoghurt

Flake the salmon, add the tomato purée and mix thoroughly. Melt the butter in a saucepan, add the flour and cook for 2 minutes. Gradually blend in the milk, bring to the boil and cook for a further 2 minutes, stirring all the time. Add sauce to the salmon, season well and stir in the dissolved gelatine and allow the mixture to cool. Add lemon juice and fold in yoghurt. Pour into a greased mould or serving dish. Chill for three hours.

Garnish with cucumber slices.

Salmon croquettes

Serves 3
1 can (194 g, 7¾ oz) pink salmon, drained
4 tablespoons breadcrumbs
1 small onion, chopped
75 g (2½ oz) low-fat margarine
30 g (1 oz) plain flour
200 ml (⅓ pint) skimmed milk
pepper

● TIP: Try adding a tablespoon of oil to the margarine, since margarine, or butter, blackens fried food very quickly.

Fry onion in 30 g (1 oz) margarine until tender – do not brown. Stir in the flour and cook for 1 minute, stirring continuously. Slowly pour in the milk and cook until thick, stirring all the time.

Stir in the salmon, pepper and add half the breadcrumbs.

Mix thoroughly and shape into six croquettes. Coat with remaining breadcrumbs and grill, turning frequently, until evenly brown.

The following selection of recipes features fish and shellfish that supply some omega-3s, but not as much as oily fish. They are a healthy choice for people who do not enjoy oily fish, as they are very low in fat and supply beneficial nutrients. A daily cod liver oil or fish oil capsule will provide your omega-3 requirement.

Prawn provençale

Serves 4

450 g (1 lb) peeled prawns (defrosted if frozen)
1 clove garlic
1 onion, chopped
120 g (4 oz) button mushrooms, sliced
30 ml (2 tablespoons) olive oil
420 g (14 oz) canned chopped tomatoes
200 ml (⅓ pint) dry white wine
salt and pepper
10 ml (1 dessertspoon) tomato purée
pinch dried mixed herbs
15 g (1 tablespoon) corn flour

Heat the oil and fry onion, garlic and mushrooms until soft. Add the tomatoes, wine, seasoning, tomato purée, herbs and simmer gently for 10 minutes.

Blend the corn flour with a little water and add to the mixture with the prawns. Stir continuously until thickened and simmer for a further 4–5 minutes.

Serve on a bed of pasta or rice with a mixed salad.

Curried halibut steaks

Serves 4

60 ml (4 tablespoons) olive oil

1 small onion, finely chopped

15 g (½ oz) fresh green and red chillies, deseeded and
sliced

2 teaspoons curry powder

½ teaspoon cumin powder

30 ml (2 tablespoons) lemon juice

4 × 225 g (8 oz) halibut steaks

salt and black pepper

Heat the oil and fry the onion and chillies with the spices
for 2–3 minutes. Add the lemon juice. Place the halibut
steaks in a shallow ovenproof dish and brush the spice
mixture over the fish. Cover and leave to marinade in the
fridge for 1–2 hours.

Place the steaks on a grill pan and grill under a moderate
to hot grill for 10–12 minutes, brushing with the remaining marinade.

Serve hot with two portions of steamed vegetables per
person.

Fish casserole

Serves 4

4 medium plaice fillets

150 g (6 oz) tomatoes, peeled and chopped

100 g (4 oz) mushrooms, chopped

20 g (4 level teaspoons) breadcrumbs

5 g (1 level teaspoon) grated lemon rind

salt and pepper

200 ml (⅓ pint) dry white wine

Mix together 60 g (2 oz) of the chopped mushrooms, bread-crumbs, lemon rind, tomato and seasoning. Place equal amounts of the mixture on the fish fillets, roll up and place in a casserole dish covering the plaice with the remaining mushrooms. Pour the dry white wine over the fish, cover and cook for 20–25 minutes at 190 °C (375 °F, mark 5).

Cod Español

Serves 4
4 cod fillets
4 slices brown bread
40 g (1½ oz) low-fat margarine
1 clove garlic, crushed
juice and grated rind of orange
salt and pepper

Place bread in blender to produce crumbs. Melt the marga-rine in a frying pan, add bread crumbs, garlic and grated orange rind. Place fish in an oiled ovenproof dish, cover with crumb mixture, season and add the orange juice. Bake at 190 °C (375 °F, mark 5).

Serve with new potatoes and green salad.

Cod with mushrooms

Serves 4
4 cod fillets
100 g (4 oz) mushrooms
1 medium onion
50 g (1½ oz) low-fat margarine

30 g (1 oz) plain flour
salt and pepper
chopped parsley (frozen parsley may be used)
skimmed milk

Skin, wash and dry the fish. Season and coat in flour. Put a sheet of aluminium foil on a baking tin and coat the centre with a little margarine. Place the fillets on the foil.

Chop the onion, slice the mushrooms and cook in a saucepan with about 30 g (1 oz) of margarine until just soft. Do not brown. Pour over the fish and fold the foil over the fish.

Cook in a preheated oven at 190 °C (375 °F, mark 5) for 30–35 minutes.

Drain the juices into a measuring jug and add sufficient milk to make a half pint. Boil for 1 minute, stirring continuously, season to taste and add the parsley. Pour the sauce over the fish.

Creamy sea fish pie

This is a creamy pie without the added calories and fat of cream, yet it still makes delicious eating.

Serves 4
300 g (10 oz) of smoked haddock fillets, skinned and cubed
300 g (10 oz) of haddock or coley fillets, skinned and cubed
30 g (1 oz) corn flour
90 g (3 oz) peas, defrosted
360 g (12 oz) can of sweetcorn, drained
freshly ground black pepper
200 ml (⅓ pint) semi-skimmed milk
90 g (3 oz) fromage frais

90 g (3 oz) wholemeal breadcrumbs
45 g (1½ oz) grated cheddar cheese (medium fat)

Preheat the oven to 190°C (375 °F, mark 5).

Place the cubed fish in a large ovenproof dish and sprinkle the corn flour over it. Stir to coat fish. Add the peas and drained corn and season with black pepper. Mix milk and fromage frais and pour over fish. Mix the breadcrumbs and cheese and spoon over fish mixture.

Bake for 25–30 minutes until topping is crisp and golden.

Serve with mixed vegetables and new potatoes.

Sole Belle Hélène

Serves 4
4 × 180 g (6 oz) sole fillets, skinned
120 g (4 oz) mushrooms, thinly sliced
1 medium onion, chopped
1 large tomato, chopped
15 ml (1 tablespoon) olive oil
salt and pepper

Preheat the oven to 150 °C (300 °F, mark 3).

Place two fillets in an ovenproof dish and cover with half the sliced mushrooms. Fry the onions and tomatoes in a little oil and place on top of the mushrooms. Add another layer of mushrooms and sandwich together with the remaining two fillets. Season with salt and pepper, cover with foil and bake for 15–20 minutes until fish is cooked.

Garnish with chopped parsley and serve with new or boiled potatoes and fresh vegetables.

Garlic prawns and scallops

Serves 2
2 scallops, sliced
225 g (8 oz) peeled prawns
15 g (½ oz) polyunsaturated margarine
1 clove garlic, crushed
1 small onion, finely chopped
salt and freshly ground black pepper

Microwave power 600–700 watt.

Melt the margarine on high for 30 seconds. Stir in the garlic and onions and cook for a further 30 seconds–1 minute. Stir in the scallops and prawns and cook covered for a further 1½ minutes, stirring after 1 minute.

Leave to stand covered for 1 minute.

Season before serving with French bread and 1 tablespoon of fromage frais spooned over.

Try these for snacks or light lunches.

Two oily fish meals a week will supply you with sufficient brain-boosting omega-3 nutrients. Vary your diet and look after your brain at other times with low-fat dishes that are high in flavour. The following non-fish dishes keep down the cholesterol and thus reduce the risk of vascular dementia.

Chicken casserole

Serves 4
4 chicken breasts, skinned

🌑 **TIP:** Almost all the fat on a chicken is under the skin, so skinning removes most of it

2 rashers smoked bacon, all fat removed
1 carrot, very thinly sliced
1 onion, chopped
1 clove garlic
180 g (6 oz) button mushrooms
1 stalk of celery, chopped
30 g (1 oz) flour
1 tablespoon mixed dried herbs
200 ml (⅓ pint) chicken stock
15 ml (1 tablespoon) tomato purée
1 small can of tomatoes
olive oil
salt and pepper

Preheat the oven to 190 °C (375 °F, mark 5).

Season the flour with salt, pepper and mixed herbs. Roll chicken breasts in the flour and brown quickly in olive oil. Transfer to a casserole dish. Add the remaining ingredients and stir to mix. Cover the casserole and bake for 1½ hours.

Serve with mashed potatoes and fresh vegetables of choice. The potatoes can be made tastier by adding chopped spring onions and cabbage, replacing butter with skimmed milk.

Lentil and bacon soup

Serves 4–6
180 g (6 oz) green lentils
200 ml (⅓ pint) chicken or vegetable stock
120 g (4 oz) smoked bacon, all fat removed, and diced

1 clove garlic
225 g (8 oz) tin of tomatoes
1 small onion, chopped
450 g (1 lb) potatoes, peeled and diced
salt and pepper

Rinse the lentils under running water and place in a large saucepan with the stock. Add tomatoes, onion, garlic, chopped bacon, salt and pepper. Bring to the boil, cover and simmer for about 1 hour or until the lentils are soft.

Add diced potatoes and cook for a further 20 minutes.

Pour into blender and purée until fairly smooth before serving.

Barbequed chicken

Serves 6
6 chicken breasts, skinned
2 small onions, peeled and chopped
15 ml (1 tablespoon) sunflower oil
5 ml (1 teaspoon) French mustard
60 g (2 oz) demerara sugar
60 ml (4 tablespoons) white wine vinegar
90 ml (6 tablespoons) tomato ketchup
30 ml (2 tablespoons) Worcester sauce

Preheat the oven to 190 °C (375 °F, mark 5).

Bake the chicken for 15 minutes, turn and bake for a further 10 minutes. Meanwhile fry the onions in oil. Mix the other ingredients and add to the onion. Bring to the boil and pour over the chicken breasts. Reduce the oven to 160 °C (310 °F). Baste the chicken with the sauce every 10 minutes until cooked.

Serve with boiled rice and salad.

The following dishes can be cooked in a microwave.

Poached salmon in white wine

Serves 2
2 salmon steaks
200 ml (⅓ pint) dry white wine
200 ml (⅓ pint) water
6 black peppercorns
1 lemon, sliced
1 bay leaf

Place the wine, water, peppercorns, lemon and bay leaf in a glass bowl. Add the salmon steaks, cover and microwave at full power for 1 minute. Turn salmon and microwave at full power for a further 1 minute.

Allow salmon to cool and serve with new potatoes and salad.

11

Planning a healthy menu

Brain health combined with happy eating – that's what this book is all about. There's no universal fix for everybody's weekly menu – we all enjoy different foods. However, expert opinion is in broad agreement on the main points regarding the dos and don'ts, and I shall concentrate on these here. The actual foods are intended as a guide only, so do feel free to modify them to suit your tastes.

A brief guide to healthy eating

Breakfast

Winter: Fruit juice (your first fruit and vegetable portion), followed by a hot cereal such as Weetabix or Quaker Oats, sweetened with a sprinkling of sultanas rather than sugar, and hot skimmed or semi-skimmed milk. Alternatively, toast lightly spread with vegetable oil, margarine or honey. Follow with a refreshing cup of good old-fashioned tea or coffee.

Once or twice a week you can enjoy a boiled egg.

Summer: Fresh fruit juice, half a grapefruit or an orange. You might make up your own cereal by adding sultanas and a handful of walnuts to a high-fibre cereal of your choice. Add cold skimmed or semi-skimmed milk.

Lunch

Sandwiches made with wholemeal bread followed by fresh fruit or yoghurt. To reduce saturated fat, choose lean meat, chicken, turkey, salad or banana fillings. Tuna sandwiches are excellent, as are pitta bread with humous and salad or the old favourite, beans on toast, which is relatively low in calories and excellent for fibre. Smoked mackerel pâté on wholemeal toast – delicious! If you use salad dressing, use a low-fat variety. Grilled sardines are quick and tasty and contain a good deal of omega-3s despite the grilling. Even better, sardines straight from the tin on toast.

Other things with which to vary your daily lunch menu include low-fat cheeses – cottage, curd, Dutch and Tendale – with some of the interesting variety of breads that are now available, lightly spread with margarine or butter.

Finish with an apple, pear or, better still, two medium tomatoes (your second portion of vegetable and fruit for the day).

● TIP: Tomatoes contain lycopene, a carotenoid that protects skin from the damaging effects of UV light, which is also related to ageing.

Dinner

Twice a week choose oily fish, where possible with Basque-style olive oil/vegetable sauce. If you can't stomach oily fish, don't worry. Eat white fish but supplement your diet with omega-3s. Twice a week choose a low-fat, non-fish recipe, such as chicken, or a tasty vegetarian dish such as ratatouille, vegetable curry, Chinese stir-fry, chunky vegetable soup with lentils or vegetarian pastas.

Twice a week choose a red meat or liver.

🔹 **TIP:** Make a point of choosing lean cuts of meat and drain off the fat by grilling or after cooking.

Enjoy chips once a week if you like, but otherwise cook potatoes in jackets, boiled or mashed. Make a point of including two vegetables, not overcooked, in large chunks rather than shredded. These are best cooked in a pressure cooker or microwave or steamed. With bread, there's a marginal benefit in eating wholemeal, wholegrain, granary or brown bread, though white is also healthy.

Don't go to extremes. Remember there are very few foods that are really bad for you. It's more a question of how much you eat. You can afford to indulge in a little cream, chocolate or, once a week with the Sunday roast, some delicious roast potatoes.

Night-time snacks

If you are trying to lose weight, plan ahead, because this is a vulnerable time when the best of intentions crumble. Keep a healthy nibble to hand, such as a bowl of mixed walnuts and raisins, to prevent mad indulgences. Alternatively, satisfy late-night hunger pangs with one of the following:

🔹 A thin slice of wholemeal bread with smoked mackerel pâté.

🔹 A slice of brown toast with honey.

- Toast with cottage cheese.

- One banana (or any other portion of fruit or vegetable).

Explanation

- Cereals for energy, fibre, calories, vitamins, and, when fortified, iron and minerals.

- Fresh fruit or fruit juice for water-soluble vitamins, including the anti-oxidant vitamin C.

- Bread for energy and vitamins, especially folic acid (important for pregnant mums!)

- Sultanas avoid the need for refined sugar.

- Walnuts really do lower cholesterol, because they contain a polyunsaturated to saturated fat ratio of 7:1, one of the highest of all foods.

- Fish for omega-3 fatty acids, vitamins D, K and A and also iron.

- Red meat or liver for iron, essential fats and vitamins.

- Margarine for essential fats and vitamins D, K and A.

- There is just as much calcium in skimmed milk as full cream, but there are few vitamins.

- The recommended amount of fat is 80g (2½ oz) a day, which should comprise at least 50 per cent unsaturates, found in vegetable and olive oils, margarine and fish, but enjoy 30 g (1 oz) of animal fat each day from meat, cream, cheeses and other dairy produce.

The total calorie requirement varies from person to person, depending on body size, gender, physical exercise, and so on. You can control your needs by varying the amount of the high-calorie foods you eat without having to exclude anything. No food is forbidden, so if you really love a food, you only need to moderate your intake and not cut it out completely.

Tip: Adding low-calorie high-fibre foods is a good way of staving off hunger pangs. If you suffer from constipation, adding lemon-flavoured Fybogel, or some other natural high-fibre alternative, is very effective, safe and adds no calories to your diet.

Putting the whole dietary advice into practice

I've given you a lot of information in this book. The advice on omega-3 intake is simple and is the single most important message, but the book should be taken as a dietary package, together with a sensible balance of unsaturated to saturated fat intake, and a reasonable amount of fibre, with the caution not to take too much salt. For some of my readers this will be ample. But I realise how hard it can be for busy people to plan a diet ahead. And for those who feel the need for some practical advice, I've drawn up two weeks of sample menus that show you how to manage healthy eating day by day.

12

Your fourteen-day planner

In setting the menu, I've given average portions, but these will vary with the normal appetite and calorie needs of readers and their families. The aim is brain health rather than weight loss, although a diet that maintains a healthy brain and mind will naturally tend to keep you at a healthy weight. I have devised as wide-ranging and interesting a menu as possible. For those who enjoy oily fish, I've provided all your omega-3 needs in this way. For those who do not enjoy oily fish, I've offered white fish or non-fish alternatives, on the assumption you will obtain your omega-3 needs with supplements.

The comments on beverages, such as tea and coffee, are limited to the first few days, so you get the idea of it. Nutritionists would advise you to confine your drinks to about four cups of tea or coffee a day and to supplement this with water or fresh fruit or vegetable juice.

Week 1

Monday

Breakfast: Fresh fruit juice or vegetable juice. Quaker Oats, made with water. Sweeten with honey or a few sultanas and add skimmed milk. Hot beverage of your choice.

Alternatively, two slices of toast, with marmalade or polyunsaturated margarine or low-fat spread. Wholemeal bread gives a better source of fibre but, if folic acid is added to the milled flour, wholemeal bread may have to be re-examined. White bread is better for pregnant women – and also for those likely to become pregnant in the near future. This is because folic acid is essential at a very early stage of pregnancy, often at the stage when women don't yet know they are pregnant.

There's nothing wrong, and a good deal right, with butter, but you should work out the saturated fat content and allow for it in your daily fat allowance.

Lunch: Tuna sandwiches, made with a high-fibre bread, followed by fresh fruit or a low-fat yoghurt.

● **TIP:** A light lunch allows you a larger family meal in the evening. If your main meal is at lunchtime, then reverse these two meals.

Tea: A cup of tea with skimmed or semi-skimmed milk. If you prefer full cream milk, allow for the saturated fat in your daily total. One bottle of full-cream milk contains more than half your daily allowance of saturated fat.

Fresh fruit, or one of the new mixed fruit drinks.

Dinner: 150 g (5 oz) lean steak, grilled, and eaten with mixed salad and a baked potato. Make a point of adding spinach to your salads (it contains lutein which offers retinal protection). But be frugal with the salad cream and dressings and choose one that is low in saturated fat. They taste just as good.

Don't be tempted to stuff the baked potato with butter. Use low-fat cottage cheese or, better still, experiment with your own dressings using natural yoghurt with mint and cucumber.

A glass of wine or fruit juice.

Dessert: There is no need to deny yourself sweet things.

Try baked apple. Core a medium-sized cooking apple, stuff with sultanas and two teaspoons of water. Prick the skin to stop it bursting and microwave for 2½ minutes on high power. Cover with foil and leave to stand for a few minutes – it will continue to bake but avoids the danger of burning your mouth.

Serve with a tablespoon of low-fat ice cream.

Follow this with a beverage of your choice.

Night-time snack: What about those dangerous little cravings late at night?

Watch the calories, of course, but try a slice of wholemeal toast with salmon pâté or smoked mackerel pâté.

Tuesday

Breakfast: As Monday, or try fresh grapefruit or a slice of pineapple, followed by your favourite cereal (containing plenty of iron) or a slice of wholemeal toast with honey.

One cup of tea or coffee.

◉ **TIP:** Pineapple contains a natural enzyme that aids digestion.

Lunch: Turkey breast sandwiches with white bread. Spread the slices very lightly with high polyunsaturated margarine. This is made easier if the margarine has been kept at room temperature long enough to soften. If you use an alternative moist filling instead of turkey, such as tinned tuna or pâté, you will need no spread at all.

Fresh fruit, such as kiwi (for lutein) or low-fat yoghurt.

Beverage of your choice.

Dinner: Sole Belle Hélène with mashed potatoes. You can cut down on the saturated fat by using skimmed milk with the potatoes instead of butter.

Serve with lashings of soft grilled tomatoes and peas.

One glass (125 ml) of white wine (optional).

Dessert: Meringue nest with fresh fruit, topped with low-fat fruit yoghurt or fromage frais.

Beverage of your choice.

Night-time snack: Fresh fruit, such as a banana. Alternatively, toast with cottage cheese, topped with a quartered tomato and a couple of slices of cucumber, seasoned with freshly ground black pepper.

Avoid tea or coffee late at night because of its caffeine content. Water, fruit juice or if you prefer to have a modest drink of alcohol last thing, take it now with a glass of water.

Wednesday

Breakfast: If you normally take fruit juice first thing, why not try a vegetable juice, like fresh tomato juice, for a change, but look out for added salt content of vegetable juices and keep to the daily salt allowance of less than 6 g.

Two Weetabix, sweetened with sultanas and hot skimmed milk.

Cup of tea.

Lunch: Kipper soup with wholemeal bread. Don't add salt but season with pepper.

Cup of tea or coffee (it's not necessary to take decaffeinated, unless for specific health reasons, if you do not drink more than 4 or 5 cups of tea or coffee a day).

Two fresh tomatoes.

Dinner: Roast chicken with new or boiled potatoes and vegetables such as broccoli and carrots.

Dessert: Strawberry Fluff – this is a special treat, easy to make and a real delight.

Pre-warm a cup by putting into a saucepan of simmering water. Dissolve one teaspoonful of gelatine in 2 teaspoons of hot water in the pre-warmed cup, which is still in the simmering water. Stir until the gelatine has dissolved. Add a little ground orange peel to a 150 g (5 oz) pot of low-fat strawberry yoghurt and stir. Add a little of this mixture to the simmering cup. Tip the cup's contents into the cold yoghurt, stirring briskly until well mixed. Leave until it begins to set.

Timing is important. At this stage, whisk the white of an egg with a pinch of salt until it starts to thicken and begins to firm. Now fold it into the strawberry mixture and mix gently before spooning into a serving dish.

Place in the fridge and leave until set.

Beverage of your choice.

Night-time snack: Try to get into the habit of taking fruit at night. As an alternative, have a breakfast cereal – try a half-portion of your favourite, with hot or cold skimmed milk.

Hot fruit juice.

Thursday

Breakfast: Kippers with a slice of wholemeal toast, followed by a refreshing glass of chilled fresh fruit juice.

Frozen kippers often come with a pat of butter in the bag. You may want to make allowance for that. Alternatively, buy kippers fresh or remove from the pack, take out the butter, and grill.

Cup of tea with skimmed milk. If you are used to full cream milk in your tea, this will take some getting used to. It might be easier to graduate through semi-skimmed or even to keep to semi-skimmed in tea. Remember that skimmed milk has all the calcium and other goodness of full cream milk without the fat.

Lunch: Fresh fruit of your choice. Tinned sardines on toast followed by mixed fruit salad, topped with natural yoghurt (optional).

Cup of tea.

Dinner: Vegetable curry.

Beverages as above.

Dessert: Fruit jelly with real fruit, such as unsweetened pine-apple, and a natural yoghurt topping. Ice cream also goes well with jelly or fruit salads and low-fat ice cream is available.

Night-time snack: A couple of handfuls of sultanas and walnuts (lower cholesterol).

Friday

Breakfast: Fresh, unsweetened fruit juice.

A boiled or poached egg with wholemeal toast (yolk contains lutein).

Lunch: Cold ham, salad and bread of your choice.

TIP: Many types of tasty and interesting bread are available – why not experiment!

Dinner: Grilled mackerel with gooseberry sauce. Serve with boiled potatoes and steamed vegetables.

Dessert: Stewed apple (or fruit of your choice) with a small portion of low-fat ice cream.

Night-time snack: Banana.

Saturday

Breakfast: Cereal with skimmed milk and sultanas. A slice of high grain or wholemeal toast with honey or marmalade.

Lunch: Smoked trout sandwiches, side salad (include spinach leaves) or low-calorie coleslaw.

Dinner: Vegetable ratatouille and white rice. This is one of my wife's recipes and one of my favourite vegetarian meals. A hit whenever we serve it to friends! Not only does it contain little saturated fat, but it includes two ingredients now thought to protect against heart attacks – olive oil and garlic. And look at all those highly coloured vegetables!

Serves 8 (but half can be frozen)
450 g (1 lb) aubergines, cubed
450 g (1 lb) courgettes, sliced

30–45 g (1–1½ oz) seasoned flour
olive oil – choose the best quality
1 bottle fruity white wine (such as Chardonnay)
225 g (8 oz) green peppers, deseeded and coarsely
    chopped
225 g (8 oz) red peppers, deseeded and coarsely chopped
450 g (1 lb) onions, coarsely chopped
450 g (1 lb) tomatoes chopped, or 1 x 397 g (14 oz) tin
4 cloves garlic, crushed
2 teaspoons sugar
1 sprig fresh or 1 teaspoon dried basil
1 tablespoon tomato purée
salt and pepper

Sprinkle the aubergines and courgettes with the seasoned flour. Heat a little olive oil in a frying pan and add the aubergines. When softened slightly, transfer to a large pan. This will leave some seasoned flour in the pan. Add 200 ml (⅓ pint) of the wine to the frying pan and stir well to incorporate the floury juices. Pour this over the aubergines. Repeat with the courgettes.

Add more olive oil to the pan and fry the peppers and onions. When softened add to the other vegetables. Place the tomatoes, garlic, sugar, basil and tomato purée in a separate pan and add a little salt and pepper. Simmer for a few minutes to reduce the liquid slightly. Rub through a sieve or liquidise briefly to give a fairly thick sauce and add it to the other ingredients. Pour in the rest of the wine and cook on the hob until vegetables are cooked but not mushy.

Skim off the olive oil, which will lie on the surface of the ratatouille. Serve with boiled rice or crusty bread.

If cooking for four, interrupt the cooking while the vegetables are still firm, take half the mixture, cool and freeze. Carry on cooking the remainder. The frozen portion can be cooked to completion at a later date.

Dessert: Another little treat – Raspberry Surprise.

Prepare and serve in 4 sundae glasses.

Into each glass place 4 raspberries to cover the bottom, 4 dessertspoons of low-fat yoghurt, 1 teaspoon runny honey. Top with a plentiful helping of raspberries.

Night-time snack: A couple of plain biscuits.

Sunday

Breakfast: If you are planning to have roast meat for dinner, why not start the day with grilled kippers, which will counter the blood fat effects of the main meal.

Put the kippers directly onto dry toast. The oil in the kippers is moist and fatty enough to avoid the need for butter or margarine.

Lunch: Crab soup with granary rolls, followed by half a small can of low-fat rice pudding with a few strawberry halves. Remember shellfish are high in omega-3s.

Dinner: Roast beef. Serve with baked potatoes (see above for stuffing the potatoes) and two vegetables, steamed in a pressure cooker or microwave. If you like gravy, choose a mix such as Bisto, which does not have added fat. However, Bisto contains salt so you do not need to add any to the cooking or to the food when served.

Enjoy a glass of red wine with the meal.

Dessert: Treat yourself to home-baked apple pie, but cut back on the pastry and use only polyunsaturated margarine. You could allow yourself a little single cream on this one day. Alternatively have low-fat ice cream or natural yoghurt.

Night-time snack: If you had turkey or salmon as your main meal, a little of this in a wholemeal sandwich.

Week 2

By now you should be getting the hang of it so I'll keep it brief.

Monday

Breakfast: Half a grapefruit, grilled, followed by two Weetabix, sprinkled with sultanas and walnuts, with hot skimmed milk.

Tea or coffee.

Lunch: Tuna and avocado salad. Dismissed as unhealthy in the anti-fat hysteria, avocados are a healthy food, high in monounsaturated fat and the beneficial carotenoid lutein. Half a medium-sized avocado adds just 100 calories to your diet, mostly unsaturated fat – compare this to the 350 calories of two fried rashers of bacon, mostly saturated fat. Glass of fruit juice.

Dinner: Turkey fillets with mushrooms served with potatoes, broccoli and carrots.

Dessert: Fresh fruit salad topped with low-fat fruit yoghurt.

Night-time snack: Toast and honey.

Tuesday

Breakfast: Natural fruit juice. Two shredded wheat with hot milk.
 Tea or coffee.

Lunch: One slice of ham and mushroom pizza with salad, followed by a fresh pear.
 Tea or coffee.

Dinner: Mackerel Portuguese served with plenty of vegetables.

Dessert: Peaches and low-calorie fruit yoghurt.

Night-time snack: Two biscuits, with a dollop of thick full-fruit jam or preserve.
 Decaffeinated coffee.

Wednesday

Breakfast: Unsweetened grapefruit juice. Poached or scrambled egg on wholemeal toast.
 Tea or coffee.

Lunch: Chicken salad. Low-fat cheese on toast or more exotic bread of your choice.

Dinner: Seafood paella. Remember that shellfish are excellent sources of omega-3s.

Dessert: Mixed seasonal fruit with low-calorie crème fraiche. You can experiment with different fruit cocktails. In season I particularly like the mix of strawberries, raspberries and blackcurrants, with beneficial levels of antioxidants that preserve brain health.

Night-time snack: Fromage frais followed by tea or fruit drink.

Thursday

Breakfast: Porridge made with water and topped with a little skimmed milk and 1 teaspoon of honey.
   Tea or coffee.

Lunch: Scrambled eggs into which you have mixed chopped smoked salmon, seasoned with black pepper and eaten with toasted wholemeal bread.

Dinner: Grilled lamb chops, boiled potatoes, peas and carrots. This is delicious with plenty of mint sauce spooned over the chops and potatoes.
   Glass of red wine.

Dessert: Apple pie and ice cream.

Night-time snack: Fresh fruit.

Friday

Breakfast: Fruit juice followed by grilled or poached kippers with a slice of wholemeal bread.
   Tea or coffee.

Lunch: Low-fat cottage cheese with plenty of mixed salad. Slice of mixed fruit teabread.

Mixed fruit teabread

This has all the richness and flavour of fruitcake, while containing virtually no saturated fat. It must be allowed to mature for 1–2 days.

180 g (6 oz) raisins
120 g (4 oz) sultanas
60 g (2 oz) currants
120 g (4 oz) soft light brown sugar
300 ml (½ pint) cold tea
1 egg, beaten
45 ml (3 tablespoons) golden syrup
225 g (8 oz) plain wholemeal flour
1½ teaspoons baking powder
½ teaspoon mixed spice

Soak the dried fruit and sugar in the tea overnight. Grease the base of a 1.6 litre (2¾ pints) loaf tin. Beat the egg and syrup into the fruit mixture. Add the flour, baking powder and spice and mix well. Spoon into the prepared tin.

Bake at 170 °C (325°F, mark 3) for 30 minutes. Cover loosely with foil and cook for 40–60 minutes until well risen and just firm. Turn on to a wire rack to cool. Wrap in foil.

Dinner: Chicken casserole.

Dessert: Meringue nest filled with strawberries or raspberries and topped with a little low-fat fruit yoghurt.

Night-time snack: Half-portion of breakfast cereal.

Saturday

Breakfast: Unsweetened fruit juice or a piece of fresh fruit. Bran flakes with skimmed milk, sweetened with chopped fruit, such as banana or prunes.

● **TIP:** If you suffer from constipation, choose prunes and caffeinated coffee – this will usually do the trick.

Tea or coffee.

Lunch: Pasta with tuna and sweet corn. Two slices of pineapple canned in its own juice.

Dinner: 180 g (6 oz) grilled pork fillet with salad and baked potatoes.

Glass of red wine.

Dessert: Strawberries topped with ice cream.

Night-time snack: Small portion of rice with jam.

Sunday

Breakfast: Fresh fruit. Grilled (not fried) streaky bacon sandwiches in wholemeal bread or toast (grilling bacon removes much of the saturated fat).

Tea or coffee.

Lunch: Roast turkey or lamb with a selection of vegetables and boiled new potatoes. (Remember to skim off the fat before making gravy.) Apple or rhubarb crumble (topping made with polyunsaturated margarine) with a little custard made with skimmed milk.

Dinner: Cold sandwich of what's left of the turkey or lamb.

Dessert: One slice of mixed fruit teabread.

Night-time snack: A slice of wholemeal bread with sandwich filling of your choice, possibly banana.

A note on calorie counting

This book is aimed primarily at maintaining brain and general body health. But obesity is a cause of ill-health, including diabetes, raised blood fats and hypertension, which in turn increase the risk of cognitive decline and dementia. So it is not unreasonable to devote a little time to helping people affected by obesity.

The problem is that all too often we are panicked into trying to lose weight too quickly. We cut back to very low-calorie intakes – for example, reducing our daily intake to less than 1,000 calories. This can lead to ill-health. Indeed, in the words of an experienced chief dietician I once worked with, 'It is virtually impossible to eat a balanced diet on less than 1,000 calories daily intake.'

Ask anybody what went wrong with their diet and most will confess that they managed to lose weight to begin with but couldn't keep to the diet for long. Any weight reduction plan must look to that more difficult long term. So let me give you a few tips based on more than 20 years' hospital experience.

* You're an individual. Your dietary needs will be different from other people's. You need to modify any weight reduction diet to suit you. The best way to do this is to start with the sort of healthy diet advocated in this book and see what happens to you over two to three weeks. If you are losing half a pound to a pound a week, you're on the right track. If you're not losing, cut the carbohydrate and fat aspects of the food by 10 per cent or so. An excellent and inexpensive calorie guide is *The Complete Calorie Counter* published by Kyle Cathie. Now give it another two or three weeks and

see what happens. Keep doing this until your weight begins to fall, slowly and steadily.

* This will lead you to discover, by trial and error, your own calorie intake on which you lose between half a pound and a pound weight per week. This will also be a diet you can stick to.

* Don't make yourself anxious by weighing yourself every day, but only weigh yourself once a week, say on Sunday mornings before breakfast, either undressed or in the same type of nightclothes.

* To help burn up calories, plan a sensible increase in your level of exercise. See the advice on physical and mental exercise in the next chapter.

13

Feeling good in mind and body

In the UK we've seen a major increase in life expectancy over the last half-century, with many of us enjoying the prospect of living longer. This is now influencing medical research and government and other funding, and more money and effort are being channelled into diseases associated with growing older. Who could object to improving our chances of staying fitter, healthier and happier into a good old age!

Sensible lifestyle strategies, including exercise, have been shown to help us maintain a healthy brain into old age.

Physical exercise

In much the same way that people erroneously assume that cognitive decline and even dementia are a natural part of getting older, they also erroneously assume that progressive physical wasting and weakening are an inevitable consequence of getting older. In fact, scientific studies have shown this to be a gross exaggeration.

Experts at the Buck Institute for Age Research, Novato, California, looked at the effects of working out on a group of 25 pensioners, with an average age of 70. They even compared them with 26 younger men and women. To start with, the older people were 59 per cent weaker, but after exercise training for six months, their strength increased so they were only 38 per cent weaker than the youngsters. The experts went on to examine what was happening at the chemical level and found objective evidence that regular exercise reverses the ageing process in the muscles.

But it didn't stop there. Researchers at the Beckman Institute at the University of Illinois showed that a regular exercise programme, even a gentle one, boosts performance in some of the key areas of the brain responsible for decision-making and mental focus. Another investigation, the Canadian Study of Health and Ageing, showed that regular physical activity appeared to protect people against age-related cognitive decline.

Others have shown similar results in dementia.

For example, Podewils and her colleagues at Johns Hopkins School of Public Health, Baltimore, looked at the lifestyles of 3,375 men and woman over the age of 65 and found that those who engaged in different types of physical activity had only half the risk of dementia of people who rarely exercised. These people didn't even go to the gym. They just did everyday chores and recreational activities such as walking, mowing the lawn and other gardening tasks, hiking, golfing, swimming and dancing.

A philosophy for any age

One of the commonest objections to taking regular exercise is the cry: 'But I'm too old, doctor!'

Now we know what to think about that! There is no age

limit to the beneficial effects of regular exercise. Fitness is a philosophy for any age. And that's a pretty good reason for thinking about exercise as well as the advice on omega-3s and diet.

Being overweight in middle age has been shown to increase the risk of dementia later in life. Exercise is also important in maintaining a healthy heart and weight. Many experts believe that part of the rise in life-threatening diseases such as heart attacks stems from the profound lifestyle changes heralded by the car and public transport. Keeping reasonably trim and fit not only boosts your self-confidence, it helps you stay sharp as you grow older. And how pleasurable and invigorating exercise can be, provided we choose an exercise that we are physically capable of and able to enjoy. We can all exercise, even people who might otherwise be relatively unfit or disabled. It just takes a little thought to work out how best to formulate an exercise programme that suits individual requirements.

I learnt a great deal from watching a group of elderly men and women perform floor exercises in a London gym – the eldest was over 90 and many suffered from arthritis or heart disease. Some even had prosthetic hip joints. What was more, they seemed to enjoy themselves tremendously. So here are a few suggestions:

- Talk to the people running your local gym and ask about sessions for your level of exercise.

- Whether you involve the local gym or plan to exercise at home, choose a programme that will stretch you a little without overdoing it.

- Find an exercise programme you *enjoy*. That way it's much more likely you'll keep to it.

- If possible, choose an exercise programme that you can do with friends. Group exercise is good company and a wonderful way of getting together for young and elderly alike. What's more, research shows that having satisfying social relationships and participating in mentally stimulating activities with others are associated with a reduced risk of cognitive decline and dementia.

Mental exercise

While regular light physical exercise helps to keep our brains and minds healthy, physical exercise may not be sufficient. Popular experience has long suggested that people who stay sharp into old age are those who take regular mental workouts, for example through doing crosswords, playing sudoku, reading and taking the trouble to maintain their knowledge base and education. As the saying goes, 'Use it or lose it!'

But what's the hard scientific evidence?

Contrary to conventional wisdom, people don't inevitably lose vast numbers of brain cells as they age. We do lose some brain cells, slowly and progressively, but research has confirmed that regular and sustained mental stimulation increases the numbers of connections between the surviving nerve cells, which counterbalances the loss of nerve cells and helps keep our minds active.

Gary Small, Professor of Ageing at the University of California, believes that regular mental stimulation really does improve mental performance as well as reducing the risk of future cognitive decline. He even has a catchy term for it: 'mental aerobics'. Timothy A. Salthouse, of the University of Virginia at Charlottesville, put it in a nutshell: 'The idea that lifestyle factors can affect both the level of cognitive functioning and the rate of age-related change in cognitive functioning is obviously very appealing because it implies that individuals can control aspects of their own destiny.'

Salthouse, who has studied the effects of mental exercise in relation to ageing in thousands of subjects, went on to make two telling observations on the effects of such mental aerobics.

The decline in some aspects of problem-solving mental ability, which starts as early as 30, is counterbalanced by an increase in accumulated knowledge – or to put it simply, experience counts. One way in which this proves invaluable is in verbal IQ. The more we practise it, the more we retain a healthy vocabulary, which can actually improve right up to retirement age. That's worth knowing. What's more, it fits with the findings that the more we exercise our brains, the more connections we form between the nerve cells.

Salthouse made another important observation. Although the mean level of problem-solving performance declines with age, that decline varies widely among individuals, with some declining very little compared to others.

The question then is this: why do some people retain better cognitive function than others? Is it just a question of having the right genes, or is it, in part, the result of differences in lifestyles, including mental aerobics? With more of us living into old age, this question is increasingly important to medical researchers.

When Joe Verghese and his colleagues at the Albert Einstein College of Medicine and Syracuse University, New York, examined this in a study of 469 subjects over the age of 75 years, they found that not only did regular physical exercise reduce the risk of dementia, so did regular mental exercise. Indeed, the best results came from the combination of regular physical *and* mental exercise, even when he allowed for base-line mental ability at the beginning of the study.

Over the last year or so, several studies have, if anything, confirmed that mental stimulation, as well as physical exercise, is a good thing, not only for improving mental function but also for reducing doctor visits, medication and falls, countering the loneliness of living alone and generally improving morale. There is even a suggestion that such exercises may slow the cognitive decline in people who are already suffering from dementia.

'But I'm just no good at fiddly things, like crosswords or sudoku!'

Don't worry! Brain exercises don't have to be difficult or daunting. Not everyone enjoys academic exercises or spending hours puzzling over a crossword or sudoku grid. Some may even think that puzzles and pastimes are a waste of time when there are jobs to be done. That's fine! Find alternative challenges. See if you can find something that looks like fun as well as being appropriate for your physical fitness and situation. How wonderful that something that engages and entertains us will also make life more interesting and varied. It might even save us from letting our brainpower slowly drain away while we slump, Homer Simpson-style, in front of the TV. What's more, if we involve friends and family, we increase the benefit. We might even encourage the happiness genie to come our way!

TIP: A good social life helps keep you young.

Here are a few suggestions you could try to see if they break up boring old routines. Some can be slotted into your daily practice, while others will take some planning to fit into your weekly schedule.

- Brush your teeth with your 'wrong' hand and take a shower with your eyes closed but with your imagination wide open.

- Change your usual route to work, the newsagent or your club. Go at a different time or on a different day. One way of measuring the quality of your brain is how it responds to change. The older we get the more set in our ways we become. Adding a little novelty is like adding spice to a dull meal.

- Memorise your shopping list. Your punishment for forgetting any item will be a return trip.

- **TIP:** Regard regular tasks like remembering a list, the words of a song or a verse of a poem as a pleasurable exercise of the 'memory organ' in your brain.

- Join the library so you can look up answers to questions that have always puzzled you. Stay curious.

- Try keeping telephone numbers in your head, but don't get too carried away with it. Keep a notebook as backup.

- Learn to speak a new language or play a musical instrument. Many people choose to learn a foreign language to help with those get-away-from-it-all winter holidays. Tackling a new subject is tough but really exercises many different 'organs' in the brain and can bring lifelong rewards.

- Join a dance class. Your brain gets an excellent workout while you're concentrating on coordinating your hands, feet and body.

- Learn to play bridge. Not only does this card game call on different parts of the brain, it has been shown to help boost the immune system. And you meet new people too.

- Surf the net. The internet opens up new ideas, skills and information to stimulate brain activity. You'll find that you can join chat groups, including people from other countries. And if you're not yet computer-literate, learning your way round a computer will keep your brain active.

- Volunteer. The number of people in the UK who volunteer is declining. If you are no longer in paid work, working to help others will force you to keep active and involved. Everybody wins.

14

Lifestyles

In the words of Ingrid Bergman, 'Happiness is good health and a bad memory.' Much as I admire the great actress, my aim is to improve your happiness and memory. The last thing I want to do is to make you more miserable by inflicting a monotonous and unappetising diet on you and your family. This is why, throughout this book, I have made it a general rule to help you not only enjoy good health, and most particularly mental health, but also to enjoy life a little more in doing so. This odyssey would be incomplete without giving you some tips on lifestyles, in particular smoking, drinking and dealing with stress, since all three are of considerable importance to your mental health and well-being.

Smoking

When asked why they smoke, smokers will claim that it steadies their nerves, or that it is one of their few personal pleasures. Unlike many of my colleagues, I refuse to be judgemental about this. Indeed, in the past I sided with smokers when colleagues and health authorities came down hard on them, even refusing them vital medical services, such as surgery, unless they kicked the habit. In those bad old days the same colleagues and health authorities did nothing at all to help smokers quit the habit – and this at a time when the tax on tobacco funded about a third of the NHS budget. Instead of criticising smokers, I set up a programme to help them, writing a manual for carers and training nurses and others to run group sessions to treat large numbers of smokers, including, in one instance, the entire workforce of a large town council. So I know pretty well what smokers go through and I remain sympathetic. Yet it is such a dangerous habit, I really would urge all smokers to quit.

Nobody can be left in any doubt that smoking is a physical and mental addiction. Even heroin users sometimes find it easier to quit the drug than to stop smoking. Yet smoking is arguably every bit as dangerous to health as heroin. Quitting is much easier these days since the NHS has adopted a more caring attitude. They now help smokers with nicotine replacement therapies and group therapy sessions.

So, if you are a smoker, you have a better chance than ever before to kick the habit. And doing so will be a major bonus for your brain. Not only is smoking associated with a high risk of heart attacks, arterial disease generally, chronic bronchitis and lung cancer, smokers also have twice the risk of non-smokers of developing Alzheimer's disease. Smoking also damages your short- and long-term memory for those everyday tasks at work and in your family and social life.

If you're still in doubt, why not discuss it with your GP or practice nurse, who will explain the help currently available and entirely free.

Alcohol

Alcohol is fine in moderation, provided you avoid driving. For many people it is part of their social culture and enjoyment. But it is definitely bad news for a healthy brain, so the alcohol measures allowed in a healthy diet are modest. Over the last two decades or so, a trend for 'super-size' wine measures has encouraged young people to consume far more than the recommended weekly allowance. According to the Office for National Statistics, the biggest increase is in young women, who are now drinking almost twice as much as they did a decade ago. But there has also been a major increase in consumption by young men. The ready availability of cheap and pleasant wines has been a major factor in this. Unfortunately, it has resulted in a dramatic, and extremely worrying, increase in serious liver disease in relatively young people.

So here are a few important facts.

You are just as likely to damage your liver with wine as with spirits or beer. And remember that, like an iceberg, alcohol is very much a hidden danger. Increasing numbers of people are presenting with advanced liver disease, even fully developed cirrhosis, by which time the damage is irreversible.

TIP: If you've overdone it with a heavy night of drinking, avoid all alcohol for at least two or three days. Your liver cells will be suffering after a binge and will take several days to recover. If you hit them with more alcohol, or worse still, further bingeing, you add to the injury without giving them the chance to recover.

So here's a general guide:

- Men should not drink more than two or three pints of beer or lager three times a week.

- Women should not drink more than two pints or the equivalent three times a week.

- It is best to take alcohol with food, because food in the gut slows down the absorption of the alcohol, lowering the blood levels and allowing more time for the liver to remove it.

- For people who already have liver disease, alcohol is absolutely forbidden.

Alcohol equivalents

The government recommends no more than 14 units a week for women and no more than 21 units a week for men. This isn't sexism. It reflects different body masses and hormonally directed alcohol susceptibilities between the two sexes.

It may come as a surprise to some people that a unit is equivalent to half a pint of beer or lager, a pub short measure of spirits or a standard (not large) pub glass of wine. Or to put it another way, a pint of beer or a *large* glass of wine hits your liver with the same punch as a double whisky.

Stress – a hidden menace

We may not realise that we are under stress. It is all too easy to get caught up with it in this modern, high-pressure age. Some will be suffering from increased irritability. They may even notice cardinal symptoms of anxiety – dry mouth, jittery legs, difficulty sleeping and lack of concentration. While this may be normal – for instance, just before a job interview or a driving test – if it describes you for long periods of time, then stress has gone way beyond what might be accepted as normal. Other tell-tale symptoms are tension headache and flying off the handle at minor upsets.

The explanation for these symptoms is very simple. Your body responds to stress by releasing adrenaline and steroids. There is even some evidence that prolonged exposure to high levels of these hormones is injurious to your brain, especially the parts of the brain involved in memory and learning.

A simple rule of thumb to determine if you are under excess stress is to ask your partner or a very close relative or friend. They can often see the signs more clearly than you can. Other common symptoms include bowel gripes, abdominal bloating, aching muscles and feeing tired most of the time, especially building up over long hours of stressful employment. If at all possible you should try to avoid stress of this nature and in particular you should avoid prolonged, or worse still, unremitting stress – there is evidence that it is harmful, causing hypertension and other problems.

Dealing with stress

In the majority of cases prolonged stress is associated with work or the home, so you can't always avoid it, but you can do a great deal about your reactions to it. I would suggest that you spend a minute or two to analyse those situations that wind you up. It's an excellent idea to get help of a partner or close friend for this. Now list those situations on a sheet of paper. In a matter of minutes you should have the causes of your personal stress in front of you.

Begin by asking yourself if you can avoid any of these situations. If the answer is yes, the remedy is obvious. If the answer is no, then try to look at the problem with a more detached perspective.

Say to yourself: 'Usually this winds me up, but I am no longer going to allow it to do so.' Take a deep breath, view the cause clearly, then take a mental step back and gauge its real importance to you. These things are often unimportant in the long run. If you don't believe me, consider what was worrying you a year ago to the day. Can you even recall it? The chances are you can't. In other words, it wasn't that important after all.

The truth of the matter is that those things that stress us out are often minor but repetitive and they can be put into a different perspective through detachment, coupled with a dose of common sense. Think of how your colleagues or family will react when in the face of such pressure you simply smile.

Other practical techniques to help you reduce stress include setting aside time during the day for relaxation, for instance with light refreshment or better still, light exercise. For many people the opportunity for light exercise will distance them from the persistent, nagging stress and it will also help reduce weight and keep the blood fats down.

Sometimes stress can be related to low self-esteem. This is not uncommon in people who are overweight or who are getting older. So let's take that mental step back and put that problem into perspective.

Think of all you've done in your life, maybe bringing

children into the world, helping others or the myriad small personal achievements that make up any individual life. Weigh the good against the bad. People are incredibly attuned to picking up vibes from others. When you think little of yourself others around you sense it and sometimes even make assumptions based on your low opinion and treat you accordingly. Don't give them the ammunition to think little of you. On the contrary, discover the zing factor in you so that your inner sun shines through.

A guide to further reading

Readers will find more information, including detailed bibliography and references, at www.swiftpublishers.com. These include key references, focusing on studies that have been cited in the text.

Introduction

Saynor, R., and Ryan, F. P. (1990). *The Eskimo Diet*. Ebury, London.

Chapter 1

Ewin, J. (2001). *Fine Wines & Fish Oil: The Life of Hugh MacDonald Sinclair*. Oxford University Press, London.

Chapter 2

Birch E. E., Birch D. G., et al (1996). Visual maturation of term infants fed omega-3 long chain polyunsaturated fatty acid (LCPUFA) supplemented formula. ARVO Meeting.

Birch, E. E., Hoffman, D. R., et al. (1998). Visual acuity and the essentiality of docosahexaenoic acid and arachidonic acid in the diet of term infants. *Pediatr Res* **44**: 201–9.

Birch, E. E., Hoffman, D. R., et al. (2002). A randomized controlled trial of long chain polyunsaturated fatty acid supplementation of formula in term infants after weaning at 6 weeks of age. *Am J Clin Nutr* **75**: 570–80.

Crawford, M. A. (2000). Placental delivery of arachidonic acid and docosahexaenoic acids: implications for the lipid nutrition of preterm infants. *Am J Clin Nutr* **71** (suppl): 1s–10s.

Helland, I. B., Smith, L., et al. (2003). Maternal supplementation with very-long-chain n-3 fatty acids during pregnancy and lactation augments children's IQ at 4 years of age. *Pediatrics* **111**: e39–44.

Helland, I. B., Saugstad, O. D., et al. (2001). Similar effects on infants of n-3 and n-6 fatty acids supplementation to pregnant and lactating women. *Pediatrics* **108**: E82.

McGregor, J. A. (2005). Omega-3 fatty acids: as important as folic acid? In *Practical Strategies to Improve Fetal and Maternal Outcomes: The Role of Omega-3 Fatty Acids Prior to Conception until after Birth*. Based on the proceedings of the Fourth Nutrition Special Interest Group at the Society of Maternal–Fetal Medicine annual meeting, 10 February 2005, Reno, Nevada. See www.obgmanagement.com.

Uauy, R., Peirano, P., et al. (1996). Role of the essential fatty acids in the function of the developing nervous system. *Lipids* **31**(Suppl): 167–76.

Williams, C., Birch, E. E., et al. (2001). Stereoacuity at age 3.5 y in children born full-term is associated with prenatal and postnatal dietary factors: a report from a population-based cohort study. *Am J Clin Nutr* **73**: 316–22.

Chapter 3

Colquhoun, I., and Bunday, S. (1981). A lack of essential fatty acids as a possible cause of hyperactivity in children. *Medical Hypothesis* **7**: 673–79.

Holman, R. T., Johnson, S. B., and Hatch, T. F. (1982). A case of human linolenic acid deficiency involving neurological abnormalities. *Am J Clin Nutri* **35**: 617–23.

Richardson, A. J., and Puri, B. K. (2000). The potential role of fatty acids in attention deficit/hyperactivity disorder (ADHD). *Prostaglandins, Leukotrienes and Essential Fatty Acids* **63**: 79–87.

Richardson, A. J., and Puri, B. K. (2002). A randomised, double blind placebo-controlled study of the effects of supplementation with highly unsaturated fatty acids on ADHD-related symptoms in children with specific learning difficulties. *Prog Neuropsycho-pharm Biol Psychiat* **26**: 233–9.

Zhang, J., Hebert, J. R., and Muldoon, M. F. (2005). Dietary fat intake is associated with psychosocial and cognitive function of school-aged children in the United States. *J Nutr* **135**: 1967–73.

Chapter 4

Beydoun, M. A., Kaufman, J. S., et al. (2007). Plasma n-3 fatty acids and the risk of cognitive decline in older adults: the atherosclerosis risk in communities study. *Am J Clin Nutr* **85**: 1103–11.

Boukje, M. v G., Tijhuis, M., et al. (2007). Fish consumption, n-3 fatty acids, and subsequent 5-y cognitive decline in elderly men: the Zutphen Elderly Study. Am *J Clin Nutr* **85**: 1142–7.

Connor, W. E. (2000). Importance of n-3 fatty acids in health and disease. *Am J Clin Nutr* **71**(suppl): 171S–175S.

Conquer, J. A., Tierney, M. C., et al. (2000). Fatty acid analysis of blood plasma in patients with Alzheimer's disease, other types of dementia, and cognitive impairment. *LIPIDS* **35**: 1305–21.

Heude, B., Ducimetiere, P., et al. (2003). Cognitive decline and fatty acid composition of erythrocyte membranes – the EVA study. *Am J Clin Nutr* **77**: 803–8.

Laurin, D., Verreault, R., et al. (2003). Omega-3 fatty acids and risk of cognitive impairment and dementia. *J of Alzheimer's Disease* **5**: 315–22.

Morris, M. C., Evans, D. A., et al. (2005). Fish consumption and cognitive decline with age in a large community study. *Arch Neurol* **62**: 1–5.

Simopolous A. P., Leaf, A., and Salem Jr, N. (1999). Essentiality of and recommended dietary intakes for omega-6 and omega-3 fatty acids. *Ann Nutr Metab* **43**: 127–30.

Whalley, L. J., Cox, H. C., et al. (2004). Cognitive ageing, childhood intelligence, and the use of food supplements: possible involvement of n-3 fatty acids. *Am J Clin Nutr* **80**: 1650–7.

Chapter 5

Andersson, C., Lindau, M., et al. (2006). Identifying patients at high and low risk of cognitive decline using Rey Auditory Verbal Learning Test among middle-aged memory clinic outpatients. *Dementia and Geriatric Cognitive Disorders* **21**: 251–9.

Barberger-Gateau, P., Letenneur, L., et al. (2002). Fish, meat, and risk of dementia: cohort study. *BMJ* **325**: 932–3.

Clark, C. M., and Karlawish, H. T. (2003). Alzheimer disease: current concepts and emerging diagnostic and therapeutic strategies. *Annals Int Med* **138**: 400–11.

Freund-Levi, Y., Eriksdotter-Jonhagen, M., et al. (2006). Omega-3 fatty acid treatment in 174 patients with mild to moderate Alzheimer disease: OmegaAD study: a randomized double-blind trial. *Arch Neurol* **63**:1402–8.

Kalmijn, S., Launer, L. J., et al. (1997). Dietary fat intake and the risk of incident dementia in the Rotterdam Study. *Ann Neurol* **42**: 776–82.

Kyle, D. J., Schaefer, E., et al. (1999). Low serum docosahexaenoic acid is a significant risk factor for Alzheimer's dementia. *Lipids* **34** (Suppl): S245.

Morris, M. C. (2006). Docosahexaenoic acid and Alzheimer disease. *Arch Neurol* **63**: 1527–8.

Ryan, F. (1996). *Virus X*. HarperCollins, London.

Ryan, F. (2007). *Between Clouds and the Sea*. Swift Publishers, UK.

Schaefer, E. J., Bongard, V., et al. (2006). Plasma phosphatidylcholine docosahexaenoic acid content and risk of dementia and Alzheimer disease. The Framingham Heart Study. *Arch Neurol* **63**: 1545–50.

Terano, T., Fujishiro, S., et al. (1999). Docosahexaenoic acid supplementation improves the moderately severe dementia from thrombotic cerebrovascular diseases. *Lipids* **34** (Suppl): S345–46.

Tully, A. M., Roche, H. M., et al. (2003). Low serum cholesterol ester-docosahexaenoic acid levels in Alzheimer's disease: a case-control study. *Br J Nutr* **89**: 483–9.

Chapter 6

Hibbeln, J. R. (2002). Seafood consumption, the DHA content of mothers' milk and prevalence rates of postpartum depression: a cross-national, ecological analysis. *J Affective Disorders* **69**:15–29.

Hibbeln, J. R., Davis, J. M., et al. (2007). Maternal seafood consumption in pregnancy and neurodevelopmental outcomes in childhood (ALSPAC study): an observational cohort study. *Lancet* **369**: 578–85.

Hibbeln, J. R., and Salam, N. (1995). Dietary polyunsaturated fatty acids and depression: when cholesterol does not satisfy. *Am J Clin Nutr* **62**: 1–9.

Marangell, L. B., Martinez, J. M., et al. (2003). A double-blind, placebo-controlled study of the omega-3 Fatty Acid docosahexaenoic Acid in the treatment of major depression. *Am J Psychiatry* **160**: 996–8.

Nemets, B., Stahl, Z., et al. (2002). Addition of omega-3 fatty acid to maintenance medication treatment for recurrent unipolar depressive disorder. *Am J Psychiatry* **159**: 477–9.

Peet, M., and Horrobin, D. F. (2002). A close ranging study of the effects of ethyl eicosapentaenate in patients with ongoing depression in spite of apparently adequate treatment with standard drugs. *Arch Gen Psychiatry* **59**: 913–19.

Raeder, M. B., Steen, V. M., et al. (2007). Associations between cod liver oil use and symptoms of depression: the Hordaland Health Study. *J of Affective Disorders* **101**: 245–9.

Chapter 7

Connor, W. E. (2000). Importance of n-3 fatty acids in health and disease. *Am J Clin Nutr* **71**(Suppl): 171S–75S.

Curtis, C. I., Hughes, C. E., et al. (1999). N-3 fatty acids specifically modulate catabolic factors involved in articular cartilage degradation. *J Biol Chem* **275**: 721–4.

Das, U. (2006). Biological significance of essential fatty acids. *JAPI* **54**: 309–19.

Geusens, P., Wouters, C., et al. (1991). Long-term effects of omega-3 fatty acid supplementation in active rheumatoid arthritis: a 12-month, double-blind, controlled study. *Arthritis and Rheumatism* **37**: 824–9.

Kremer, J. M. (1997). Omega-3 fatty acid supplements in rheumatoid arthritis. *ISSFAL Newsletter* **4**: 5–8. (An important summary of the American findings.)

Kremer, J. M., Jubiz, W., et al (1987). Fish-oil fatty acid supplementation in active rheumatoid arthritis: a double-blind, controlled, crossover study. *Ann Int Med* **106**: 497–502.

Lau, C. S., Morley, K. D., and Belch, J. J. F. (1993). Effects of fish oil supplementation on non-steroidal anti-inflammatory drug requirements in patients with mild rheumatoid Arthritis – a double-blind placebo controlled study. *Br J Rheumatology* **32**: 982–9.

Lichtenstein, A. H., Allel, L. J., et al. (2006). Diet and lifestyle recommendations revision 2006: a scientific statement from the American Heart Association Nutrition Committee. *Circulation* **114**: 82–6.

Marchioli, R., Barzi, F., et al. (2002). Early protection against sudden death by n-3 polyunsaturated fatty acids after myocardial infarction: time-course analysis of the results of the Gruppo Italiano per lo Studio dell Sopravvivenze nell'Infarcto Miocardi (GISSI)-Prevenzione. *Circulation* **105**: 1897–1903.

Simopoulos, A. P. (2002). Omega-3 fatty acids in inflammation and autoimmune diseases. *J Am College of Nutrition* **21**: 495–505.

Chapter 8

Yehuda, S. (2003). Omega-6/omega-3 ratio and brain-related functions. In Simopoulos, A. P. and Cleland, L. G. (eds.) *World Rev Nutr Diet* **92**: 37–56.

Yehuda, S., Rabinovitz, S., and Mostofsky, D. I. (2005). Essential fatty acids and the brain: from infancy to aging. *Neurobiol. Aging* **26** (Suppl): S98–102.

Yehuda, S., Rabinovitz, S., et al. (2002). The role of polyunsaturated fatty acids in restoring the aging neuronal membrane. *Neurobiol. Aging* **23**: 843–53.

Chapter 9

Berr, C. (2000). Cognitive impairment and oxidative stress in the elderly: results of epidemiological studies. *Biofactors* **13**: 205–9.

Deschamps, V., Barberger-Gateau, P., et al. (2001). Nutritional factors in cerebral aging and dementia: epidemiological arguments for a role of oxidative stress. *Neuroepidemiology* **20**: 7–15.

Dye, L., and Lluch, A. (2000). Macronutrients and mental performance. *Nutrition* **16**: 1021–34.

Gonzalez-Gross, M., Marcos, A., et al. (2001). Nutrition and cognitive impairment in the elderly. *Br J Nutr* **86**: 313–21.

Hepburn, F. N., Exler, J., and Weihrauch, J. L. (1986). Provisional tables on the content of omega-3 fatty acids and other fat components of selected foods. *J Am Diet Assoc* **86**: 788–93.

Jama, J. W., Launer, L. J., et al. (1996). Dietary antioxidants and cognitive function in a population-based sample of older persons. *Am J Epidemiol* **144**: 275–80.

Masaki, K. H., Losonczy, K. G., et al. (2000). Association of vitamin E and C supplement use with cognitive function and dementia in elderly men. *Neurology* **54**: 1265–72.

Sies, H., and Stahl, W. (2004). Carotenoids and UV protection. *Photochem Photobiol Sci* **3**: 749–52.

Sies, H., and Stahl, W. (2004). Nutritional protection against skin damage from sunlight. *Ann Rev Nutr* **24**: 173–200.

Chapter 10

Solfrizzi, V., Panza, F., et al. (1999). High monounsaturated fatty acids intake protects against age-related cognitive decline. *Neurology* **52**: 1563–9.

Chapter 12

Cathie, K. (1976). *The Complete Calorie Counter.* Pan Books, London.

Chapter 13

Arkin, S. (2007). Language-enriched exercise plus socialization slows cognitive decline in Alzheimer's disease. *American Journal of Alzheimer's Disease and Other Dementias* **22**: 62–77.

Cohen, G. D., Perlstein, S., et al. (2006). The impact of professionally conducted cultural programs on the physical health, mental health and social functioning of older adults. *The Gerontologist* **46**: 726–34.

Gatz, M. (2005). Educating the brain to avoid dementia: can mental exercise prevent Alzheimer's disease? *PLoS Medicine* **2**: 38–40.

Laurin, D., Verreault, R., et al. (2001). Physical activity and risk of cognitive impairment and dementia in elderly persons. *Arch Neurol* **58**: 498–504.

Melov, S., Tarnopolsky, M. A., et al. (2007). Resistance exercise reverses aging in human skeletal muscle. PLoS, issue 5, e465. Published on line.

Podewils, L. J., Guallar, E., et al. (2005). Physical activity, *APOE* genotype, and dementia risk: findings from the cardiovascular health cognition study. *Am J Epidemiology* **161**: 639–51.

Salthouse, T. A. (2006). Mental exercise and mental ageing. *Perspectives on Psychological Science* **1**: 68–87.

Stine-Morrow, E. A. L., Parisi, J. M., et al. (2007). An engagement model of cognitive optimization through adulthood. *The Journals of Gerontology Series B: Psychological Sciences and Social Sciences* **62**: 62–9.

van Praag, H., Kempermann, G., and Gage, F. H. (2000). Neural consequences of environmental enrichment. *Nature Reviews: Neuroscience* **1**: 191–8.

Verghese, J., and Lipton, R. B. (2003). Leisure activities and the risk of dementia in the elderly. *NEJM* **348**: 2508–16.

Weuve, J., Kang, J. H., et al. (2004). Physical activity, including walking, and cognitive function in older women. *JAMA* **292**: 1454–61.

Wilson, R. S., Bennett, D. A., et al. (2003). Cognitive activity and cognitive decline in a biracial community population. *Neurology* **61**: 812–16.

Wilson, R. S., Mendes de Leon, C. F., et al. (2002). Participation in cognitively stimulating activities and risk of incident of Alzheimer's disease. *JAMA* **287**: 742–8.

Where to go for support

People who need advice on alcohol or smoking cessation should speak in confidence to their GP or practice nurse. There are helpful government initiatives, often organised through the local Primary Care Trust, which offer free help. The same advice applies to people seeking advice for any of the conditions discussed in this book.

The following organisations will also provide help and support:

Dementia UK, published in 2007, is available from the Alzheimer's Society, Gordon House, 10 Greencoat Place, London SW1P 1PH. This society, which has branches throughout the UK, supports research and other initiatives for sufferers and their carers.

You can contact the Alzheimer's Society by: phone 020 7306 0606, Fax 020 7306 0808 or e-mail enquiries@alzheimers. org.uk. Or visit the society online at http://www.alzheimers.org. uk.

For help with depression and other mental disorders, visit www.mind.org.uk. The Mind information line (0845 766 0163) is open Monday–Friday, 9.15 am–5.15 pm.

Colleagues and other healthcare workers wanting to know more about the scientific evidence, or needing advice on any of the aspects in this book should visit the Brain Food Diet pages at www.swiftpublishers.com.

Other useful sources of information

Alzheimer's disease and prevention: http://www.yourhealthbase.com/Alzheimer's_Prevention.htm

The Avon study, Children of the 90s: http://www.alspac.bris.ac.uk/welcome/index.shtml

The British Nutrition Foundation: http://www.nutrition.org.uk

Exercise and prevention of cognitive decline: http://www.beckman.uiuc.edu/news/synergy/SynergySpring2007.pdf http://www.news.uiuc.edu/II/03/0306/0306.pdf

Food Standards Agency – an independent organisation that monitors healthy eating in the UK: http://www.eatwell.gov.uk/

A medical overview of omega-3s in pregnancy and infancy: http://www.obgmanagement.com/mededlibr/PDFs/0605_THR-O-5.pdf

Memory test for early diagnosis of dementia: http://ki.se/ki/jsp/polopoly.jsp?d=130&a=33885&l=en&newsdep=130

MIND fact sheet on depression: http://www.mind.org.uk/Information/Factsheets/Statistics/Statistics per cent207.htm

The Nun Study into ageing and Alzheimer's disease: www.mc.uky.edu/nunnet/

Omega-3s in dyslexia, dyspraxia, ADHD and autism: http://www.dyslexic.org.uk/docs/AJR_Nutrition_Practitioner-FA per cent20in per cent20DDAA03.doc

Omega-3s in psychiatric disorders: http://www.groupadpsych.org/files/2003/omega3.pdf

Overview of omega-3s and cancer: http://www.ahrq.gov/clinic/epcsums/o3cansum.htm

The Vegetarian Society of the United Kingdom: http://www.vegsoc.org

World Health Organisation – prevention of mental disorders: http://www.who.int/mental_health/evidence/en/prevention_of_mental_disorders_sr.pdf

A few important terms

Age-related cognitive decline, or ARCD – a condition in which there is impairment of memory and cerebral function associated with ageing, sufficient to interfere with the normal pattern of life.

ALA – alpha-linolenic acid, an essential omega-3 fatty acid.

Alzheimer's disease – the most common form of dementia, characterised by a characteristic pathology in the brain, with so-called amyloid plaques.

ARA – arachidonic acid, an omega-6 fatty acid. This is readily formed in the body from dietary linoleic acid, or LA.

Dementia – the loss of memory and other cognitive powers at any age in someone who formerly had normal mental function. It includes a number of causes and patterns of disease, but the majority are caused by Alzheimer's disease or vascular dementia.

DHA – docosahexaenoic acid, an omega-3 fatty acid.

EPA – eicosapentaenoic acid, an omega-3 fatty acid.

Essential fats – fatty acids that are important for normal health. These include linoleic acid (LA), which is converted to arachidonic acid (ARA) in the body, and alpha-linolenic acid (ALA), which has some potential for conversion to eicosapentaenoic acid (EPA) and docosahexaenoic acid (DHA), which are only found in substantial amounts in oily fish, shellfish and certain algae.

Monounsaturated fatty acid – a fat in which there is one double stranded joint (chemical double bond) along the string of carbon beads that make up a fatty acid.

Omega-3 – a PUFA in which the first double stranded joint (chemical double bond) is on the third carbon from the omega end of the chain. Examples include docosahexaenoic acid (DHA), eicosapentaenoic acid (EPA) and alpha-linolenic acid (ALA).

Omega-6 – a PUFA in which the first double stranded joint (chemical double bond) is on the sixth carbon from the omega end of the chain. Examples include linoleic acid (LA) and arachidonic acid (ARA).

Omega-9 – a fatty acid in which the first double stranded joint (chemical double bond) is on the ninth carbon from the omega end of the chain. Oleic acid (from olive oil) is a monounsaturated omega-9 fatty acid.

PUFA, or polyunsaturated fatty acid – a fat in which there are two or more double stranded joints (chemical double bonds) along the string of carbon beads. All of the fats essential to human health are PUFAs.

Saturated fat – a fat in which there are no chemical double bonds.

Vascular dementia – dementia caused by arterial disease to the brain.

If you have a query or suggestion about any aspect of *The Brain Food Diet*, please write to me at

frankryan@swiftpublishers.com

Please ensure that you put 'the Brain Food Diet' in your title or subject line, since I receive hundreds of emails a day, most of which are removed by spam filters.

Be happy, be healthy!

Dr Frank Ryan